MW00324592

Doing Relationship-Centred Dementia Care

of related interest

Timely Psychosocial Interventions in Dementia Care
Evidence-Based Practice
Edited by Jill Manthorpe and Esme Moniz-Cook
Foreword by Helen Rochford-Brennan, Chairperson of the
European Working Group of People with Dementia
ISBN 978 1 78775 302 0
eISBN 978 1 78775 303 7

Promoting Resilience in Dementia Care
A Person-Centred Framework for Assessment and Support Planning
Julie Christie
Forewords by Wendy Mitchell and Mary Marshall
ISBN 978 1 78592 600 6
eISBN 978 1 78592 601 3

Namaste Care for People Living with Advanced Dementia
A Practical Guide for Carers and Professionals
Nicola Kendall
Foreword by Joyce Simard
ISBN 978 1 78592 834 5
eISBN 978 1 78450 975 0

Communication Skills for Effective Dementia Care
A Practical Guide to Communication and Interaction Training (CAIT)
Edited by Ian Andrew James and Laura Gibbons
ISBN 978 1 78592 623 5
eISBN 978 1 78592 624 2

Embracing Touch in Dementia Care
A Person-Centred Approach to Touch and Relationships
Luke Tanner
Foreword by Danuta Lipinska
ISBN 978 1 78592 109 4
eISBN 978 1 78450 373 4

DOING RELATIONSHIP-CENTRED DEMENTIA CARE

David I.J. Reid

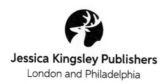

Jessica Kingsley Publishers
London and Philadelphia

First published in Great Britain in 2021 by Jessica Kingsley Publishers
An Hachette Company

1

Copyright © David Reid 2021

All rights reserved. No part of this publication may be reproduced, stored
in a retrieval system, or transmitted, in any form or by any means without
the prior written permission of the publisher, nor be otherwise circulated
in any form of binding or cover other than that in which it is published and
without a similar condition being imposed on the subsequent purchaser.

A CIP catalogue record for this title is available from the
British Library and the Library of Congress

ISBN 978 1 78592 306 7
eISBN 978 1 78450 613 1

Printed and bound in Great Britain by Clays Ltd

Jessica Kingsley Publishers' policy is to use papers that are natural,
renewable and recyclable products and made from wood grown in
sustainable forests. The logging and manufacturing processes are expected
to conform to the environmental regulations of the country of origin.

Jessica Kingsley Publishers
Carmelite House
50 Victoria Embankment
London EC4Y 0DZ

www.jkp.com

For my beautiful children, Lola, Hannah and Jasper

Dedicated to the life and memory of Hetty Reid

Contents

Contents

Preface

For me, dementia is personal.

Anyone who writes about dementia does so from their own perspective, drawing on their unique experiences and driven by a sense of purpose. A number of things bother me about current approaches to dementia care and support, and here are two to start. It bothers me that dementia care and support practitioners, who advocate this or that approach in dementia care and support, often paint themselves out of the scene. The most bothersome are those individuals who claim to be using, for example, a 'person-centred', 'relationship-centred' or 'anything-centred' approach while being unable to explain what they actually mean by this and are unable to indicate from where these ideas originate. If you can't explain what you are doing and why in dementia care and support, then how can you justify your approach?

It also bothers me when some suggest that excellence in dementia care and support is 'intuitive', that you'll 'get it', a lightbulb moment, if you follow the invocations of the latest 'dementia guru'. If you don't 'get it' then you simply were not listening hard enough. I have a zero tolerance towards anyone who claims to possess the 'truth' about dementia care and support because, invariably, the discussion must lead back to the self-proclaimed dementia guru and their apparent brilliance.

Neither of these positions is satisfactory. This is because, in each, the dementia care and support practitioner must consider themselves, or is considered by others, to be no more than a cipher for superior knowledge. So, I want to be open at the start about my perspective and also make it clear that I consider myself to be simply one person among many who may have something useful to contribute to thinking about dementia care and support.

I do not have a diagnosis of dementia, but during the last 27 years I have met and worked with many people who have, along with their family members, and a wide range of dementia care and support practitioners. I have met people while undertaking academic research, when employed as a development worker for a UK dementia charity and, more recently, in the role of a university teacher. However, there is absolutely no doubt in my mind that it is those who have dementia, those who provide support to family members or friends who have dementia and those who work to support persons with dementia and their families whose expertise is most valuable and most in need of being heard. Collectively, you are the dementia experts.

The reason I believe this is because the core of my own dementia education is informed by what I have learned from those affected by dementia and people who support those with and affected by dementia. However, I am happy to own any shortcomings in my understanding of dementia care and support made evident in this book. I am still learning, after all. On reflection, I can identify some specific encounters which have undoubtedly had a significant impact on my thinking – and sharing these here is a way of demonstrating how dementia is personal to me. It follows that these encounters indicate how and why I have come to view a relationship-centred approach as most suitable for promoting excellence in dementia care and support.

The idea of providing a neat and tidy account of my significant influences might be seductive but it's bound to be inaccurate.

Accounts from memory are all imperfect, and are organised, knowingly or otherwise, to serve the audience being addressed. The reasons for dwelling on my perspective, my experiences and my sense of purpose are indicated at the start. In order to engage in critical debate about dementia care and support I believe that contributors must be open and honest about where their ideas originate, about what principles they are wedded to, and why. Once this task is out of the way, the reader will have a better idea of what I mean when I refer to a relationship-centred approach and why I have come to believe this is a useful device for promoting excellence in dementia care and support.

My great-grandmother, Hetty Reid, had dementia. I was 12 years old when she died and it was at that point the word 'dementia' entered my vocabulary. I didn't know Hetty well but I had met her a few times at her flat. She was a friendly and kind woman. The impact of her death on my mum was devastating. When my mum had been a teenager, she had gone through a period of estrangement from her own parents and had gone to live with Hetty for a while. In my mum's and others' recollection, Hetty had been an incredible woman. Apparently, she had been a fixture of her East End community during the war, available at all hours to help others, be this tending to people who had died or sharing her telephone with anyone needing to use it. She'd wring the necks of chickens in her small yard and what she couldn't bake in her rudimentary oven wasn't worth eating. More importantly, she'd cared about my mum and listened to her. Hetty's death introduced me to dementia and its impact within families.

In 1992, as a second-year undergraduate at Royal Holloway and Bedford New College, I was President of the Geographical Society. One of my roles involved arranging an external speakers' programme and I was very pleased when Professor Mike Oliver agreed to come and speak. At best, I had probably skim-read a couple of chapters of *The Politics of Disablement* (Oliver, 1990) but had been struck, as many are, by the shift in emphasis it suggests from blaming individuals for their disability to instead seeking explanations for disability in structural forms.

After his talk, I thanked Professor Oliver and proceeded to impose on him some ideas I had for my dissertation. Our cohort had recently returned from a field trip to Majorca where a friend and I had spent some time thinking about the problems facing tourism officials seeking to market Palma as a winter holiday destination for 'the elderly'. We had noticed and then mapped the number of businesses with stepped access within a small zone of the city. Overwhelmed by my cleverness, I suggested to Professor Oliver that I was thinking of focusing my dissertation research on the lived experience of disabled people. He uttered an expletive in his response, suggesting that I build my career 'on the backs of some other poor unfortunates'. Mike's pointed response introduced me to the political dimensions of self-advocacy and prompted me, sharply, to think a lot more about whose voices are heard in research studies and, more generally, in society.

A few years later I was based at the University of Stirling but conducting fieldwork for my Master's dissertation in a day-care setting in south London. By this time, I was reading the dementia care and support literature and had decided to explore which of three data collection approaches would be most effective for 'hearing the voices of people with dementia': structured questionnaires, semi-structured questions, unstructured questions (Reid, 1996). I spent a lot of time with Harry, a day-care service user. In our unstructured conversations, he told me a bit about his life. His narrative would sometimes meander as much as the bike rides he told me he used to go on with friends to Brighton when he was a young man. He'd be telling me about cycling to Brighton, then about 'meeting girls', then about his wife and his family, then about working for Hansard as a printer.

It was during one of these conversations that Harry went

back to talking about working nights as a printer, about how the mechanised binding process involved, first, folding the paper, before the machine would then 'clitch' it into the spine of the Hansard journal. Until then, I had been focused on the range of biographical information that Harry communicated in these kinds of interactions, and enjoying our conversations. Later, at home, I looked up the word 'clitch' in the family dictionary and found that it meant 'to cause to adhere'. Harry had taught me a new word but there was no immediate epiphany. It was a few years later that I looked back and realised that learning a new word from Harry symbolised something really important about the origin of knowledge in discussions of dementia care and support. I connected it to what Professor Oliver had said. The result was that I started to view my own role as a researcher, and then, later, as an educator, much more critically.

A further significant influence was what I learned working with Colin Ward between 2014 and 2018. Sadly, Colin died in 2019 after a short illness following several years living with posterior cortical atrophy (PCA) and Alzheimer's disease. Before his retirement, Colin was a senior civil servant within local government, and when I met him and his wife, Irene, through his son-in-law Nick, he told me he was keen to maintain a sense of purpose and spread the word about PCA, a type of dementia which is relatively unknown.

Colin was already involved with PCA research studies (National Institute for Health Research, 2017) when I met him, and he generously accepted my invitation to come and speak about his experiences of living with dementia to university students. As we lived close to each other, we caught the same train on the days he would journey from Hull to stand up and speak in front of either postgraduate or undergraduate students about how his and Irene's lives had changed. Despite Colin's unfamiliarity with this kind of work, he proved to be a natural at teaching. He prepared lists of topics to cover in advance. Like any good teacher, he had a clear idea of content and learning outcomes. Watching him and the students in whichever classroom or the lecture theatre we were in, I could think of nothing more inspiring and valuable than persons with dementia like Colin educating the next generation of dementia care leaders and health care practitioners. Colin told me he got a thrill from teaching, not least because he was actively engaged in raising awareness of PCA. I've since reflected a number of times – in fact, as I type these very words – that if Colin could stand up and speak, I could eventually finish writing this book.

* * *

This book focuses on the key typical interpersonal relationships that characterise the practical work of dementia care and support. A series of arguments are made at different points, and summarised in the conclusion, for how a better understanding of these relationships can provide intelligence about how to make the most of them and, in so doing, drive up the quality of that care and support for everyone.

Throughout the following chapters, I encourage you to reflect on your own care or support setting and the questions that you bring with you to your reading of this text. The book is aimed at dementia care and support practitioners of one type or another, people working in health or social care roles or in the voluntary sector, and the content is deliberately geared to this audience.

However, I hope that persons with dementia and family members or friends will find useful ideas and/or things to disagree with or contest in what I suggest here. The most important thing is that we're now talking much more about dementia than we used to. So many steps forward have been taken in recent years, with persons with dementia in the vanguard of innovation and change. In my view, this momentum must be maintained so that all those affected by dementia can expect as standard, and not as an exception, the continuation of meaningful and valued lives. I hope that self-professed allies like me have a role to play, while remaining vigilant of the danger of professing to speak for those who know best.

In Chapter 1, the building blocks of a relationship-centred approach are described. An attempt is made to provide some orientation to the typical interpersonal relationships that tend to occur in dementia care and support, and a rationale for this focus is provided. The identification of the key partners – individuals with dementia, family members or friends, and care practitioners – is accompanied by ideas about how their experiences of dementia must vary. Suggestions are made about how to reconsider the value of these relationships beyond what is implied by the superficial labels that are often ascribed to each. A case is made for giving each set of experiences equal weight in discussions of dementia care and support while also asserting that the care or support practitioner has a special responsibility to ensure this occurs. It is also argued that an orientation towards learning should accompany care and support practitioners' interactions with persons with dementia, family members and supporters.

Chapter 2 focuses on the first of the three key partners in relationship-centred dementia care and support: persons with dementia. This chapter offers an introduction into some of the things that have been learned about the experiences of some persons with dementia from research and consultation, including from my own research. I argue for the adoption of a critical approach to all claims of dementia knowledge. In particular, I suggest it is vital that a critical view is applied to knowledge claims associated with attempts to understand the perspectives of persons with dementia, pointing to the impact that the methods used to obtain this information can have on what is learned, as well as the seeping-in of others' agendas when decisions are made about what to research. The aim is to suggest some simple strategies you can adopt to improve your understanding of the experiences of persons with dementia, one at a time, where you work, and to engage persons with dementia as experts in order to enhance service quality.

Chapter 3 focuses on learning from the experiences of family members and friends of persons with dementia. As they are the second key partner in a relationship-centred approach to dementia care and support, it is argued that the category 'family members and supporters' typically contains a wide range of different individual perspectives, all of which deserve recognition and attention from the care and support practitioner. As well as identifying some of the distinctive support needs of family members and friends, emphasis is placed on the ongoing nature of the relationships these people have with people who have dementia. To assist with this, Jane Watson provides an account of her father, James. Finally, it is argued that families and friends possess potentially invaluable sources of expertise and insight. Some ways in which care practitioners can access this expertise in practice, for mutual benefit, are suggested.

The third partner in the approach to care and support outlined here is the care and support practitioner. In Chapter 4, having considered the value of learning from the experiences of persons with dementia and their families and supporters, the spotlight shifts to practitioners and their experiences of dementia. How do practitioners experience dementia? It might be a stretch to suggest that dementia care practitioners' full humanity is rarely acknowledged, yet they are the ultimate influencers of dementia care and support but remain bafflingly undervalued. In this chapter, it is argued that there is an under-recognised complexity to dementia care and support. Consequently, a lack of respect and seriousness is attributed to the perspectives of those who actually 'do' dementia care on a daily basis. Practitioners are encouraged to reflect on their practice as a regular part of their work. However, it is argued that there is a real need for honesty about a range of issues.

In Chapters 5–7, the focus on care and support practitioners' experiences sharpens to examine personal experience, comprising private, public and practical experiences. In Chapter 5, private experiences of dementia are discussed and examples are drawn on to suggest that imaginative and creative methods, such as engagement in art and music, offer practitioners productive routes by which to explore their private experiences of dementia and, thereby, understand their own perspectives more clearly and authentically. By extension, it is suggested that private experiences influence the interpersonal communication that practitioners engage in with persons with dementia and their families and friends.

The idea that care and support practitioners have practical experiences of dementia is developed further in Chapter 6. It is suggested that, in case they do not realise it, practitioners are very much part of a wider dementia community. To examine what care and support practitioners might do to seek improvements in practice, Alison Gordon's concept of the 'dementia passionista' and Natasha Wilson's ideas about a 'dementia tribe' are introduced. The 'team' or practice community practitioners work with every day is argued to represent an important shared resource and has its place within a relationship-centred approach. Suggestions are made about the practitioners' membership of other dementia communities of practice and the potential they offer for sharing and gaining peer expertise.

In Chapter 7, the central argument that the expertise of dementia care and support practitioners is crucial to dementia care and support is contrasted with assumptions in dementia service standards and recommendations for dementia training and education in the UK. It is shown that current approaches in dementia care education seem only to tell practitioners what to know, do not acknowledge the expertise such people possess, offer nothing in terms of suggesting the most effective ways to learn, and do not acknowledge that practitioners work within organisations. It is argued that this situation needs to change, with one route being greater participation of practitioners in these communities; ideas about the direction to take to achieve this are given.

The key components of this critical, relationship-centred approach to dementia care and support are summarised in Chapter 8. There are a number of distinctive features to the approach but also a number of identifiable steps to *doing*, to action, to making a difference. Unlike other approaches, this one puts dementia care and support practitioners in the foreground, alongside persons with dementia and family members and friends. The notion of a 'University of Dementia' is outlined as a route forward which would value the true experts in dementia care and support. Some limitations in my approach are identified and readers are encouraged to contact me with any others they spot. As noted earlier, I am learning, too. It should be clear by now that this book is not in any way intended to be the last word on dementia care and support; how could it be? I hope that it represents an interesting and useful contribution to the ongoing conversation.

David Reid

■ CHAPTER 1 ■

Introducing a Critical, Relationship-Centred Approach to Dementia Care and Support

One of the biggest challenges faced by persons with dementia on a daily basis is that of uncertainty. A sense of uncertainty can also affect practitioners, that is, wanting to offer appropriate support or care but being unsure where to start and how to go about doing this. One way forward is to try and create a productive, fair and empowering space for consideration of these questions. I believe this can be achieved by focusing on the interpersonal relationships which practitioners develop with persons with dementia, their families and supporters, as they offer care and support.

This way of thinking encourages practitioners to recognise the significant role and impact they have in determining what gets called 'dementia care and support'. With a credible framework to provide scaffolding for this inquiry, through reflection and gentle critical thought, practitioners can become increasingly self-aware. By becoming so, they will not just avoid inadvertently defaulting to the so-called 'biomedical model of dementia' – an ever-present danger in imagining dementia care and support – but they will understand better the benefits of collaboration with persons with dementia and their families or supporters, of taking practical steps together, towards a more meaningful way of practising dementia care and support.

A vital first step is to begin to – and then get into the habit of continuing to – question what the biomedical model suggests is the 'truth' about dementia and its relevance to care and support. Indeed, this first step should be followed by the development and adoption of a critical stance towards all dementia knowledge. It might sound like a big ask but it's not at all difficult and it bears early fruit. Questioning claims about dementia that arise from the biomedical model is the first action required. At this point, it helps to reflect on what use of the term 'biomedical' actually implies in relation to branches of dementia knowledge. The term is defined as relating to biomedicine, biology and medicine (Merriam-Webster [online], 2020). Therefore, neuroscientists who are engaged in seeking to understand what causes the pathology associated with dementia do so to advance biochemical or biological knowledge. Based on advances in biological understanding, they also seek to develop treatments for dementia or interventions to protect against the development of dementia. Undoubtedly, this worldwide scientific endeavour represents the best chance we have of, in some way, 'defeating' dementia.

Biomedical also refers to medicine, which has been defined as 'the art or science of prevention, diagnosis and cure of disease' (Chambers Dictionary, 2003). This definition brings into focus those who have the medical training to undertake these tasks when the disease (or, more appropriately, syndrome) is dementia. These professionals are typically neurologists, neuropsychologists, geriatric psychiatrists and geriatricians and they have distinctive aims and objectives that come with their roles.

In order to understand dementia biomedically, and to become proficient in their roles, these professionals require specialist education. Consequently, their understandings of dementia range from the microscopic, cellular level, to the physiological and behavioural symptoms of cellular changes in individual human beings, to the knowledge to be able to apply and interpret standardised protocols for diagnostic testing. The biomedical model of dementia and its associated language and terminology originates in and guides the work of these expert professionals (see e.g. Berrios, 1990). A practical result of their work – people with a formal diagnosis of dementia – brings a wide range of dementia care and support practitioners into the picture. However, dementia care and support practitioners do not do the same work as neuroscientists or neurologists, so should they be using the same biomedical approach, including the same language and terminology, despite this being what defines a 'person with dementia'?

Neurologists and fellow qualified professionals use a range of standardised methods to determine whether someone has a diagnosis of dementia, and this includes assessing a person's symptoms. In the UK, triggered by a referral from a GP, this typically takes place in multi-disciplinary National Health Service (NHS) memory clinics or by specialists in their respective departments. For dementia care and support practitioners, the specialists that encounter persons with dementia after their diagnoses, the language of symptoms and the attribution of symptoms to brain pathology offer information about dementia that is simultaneously both potentially very useful but also potentially very damaging. The way for dementia care practitioners to avoid the potentially damaging use of this kind of dementia information is to recognise clearly and unambiguously that they have a hugely different role to perform in dementia care and support from that of medical practitioners.

Once this is recognised it is just a short step to becoming more critical consumers of dementia knowledge and, vitally, to begin to view expertise in their domain as residing with those with whom they are involved on a daily basis in dementia care and support, and with themselves.

A biomedical approach to dementia offers a vital understanding of what 'it' is, how to diagnose it, what might be done pharmacologically to reduce its catastrophic effects and, it is hoped, one day offer protection or cure. While this model has dominated our understanding since dementia was first studied by biomedical scientists, this dominance should not be taken to mean that biomedical knowledge can or should also determine the best ways to offer dementia care and support. It's just that it has and still does, despite what is now 30 years since the push-back against it began, when alternative ideas about dementia and dementia care and support, including those authored by persons with dementia and their supporters, began to emerge. While it would be hard to find anyone who does not want to 'defeat dementia', the art and science of dementia care and support is fundamentally about *accepting* dementia, and thereby *valuing* the ongoing lives of people diagnosed with dementia and the lives of their significant others.

There is more on the rejection of the biomedical model of dementia for care and support in Chapter 2. However, it is vitally important for care practitioners to realise that they each have *a choice* to make about what dementia knowledge to draw on in their practice.

It is easy to become a critical consumer of dementia knowledge and now is the time to begin. It is as simple as adding your own question marks to claims that are made about dementia. The impact is immediate, turning seemingly authoritative statements of fact into legitimate topics for discussion and further investigation. Some statements I have heard frequently expressed by dementia care and support practitioners include:

'people with dementia live in the past'; 'wandering is a symptom of dementia'; 'people with dementia can become violent'; 'they don't understand'. Turning these into questions, by adding a question mark, initiates discussion about whether these are indeed symptoms of dementia – living in the past, wandering, violence (or 'challenging behaviour') and lacking understanding. I return to these specific questions later on in the chapter.

When you investigate the 'symptoms of dementia', one of the first things that can strike you is how many 'types' of dementia exist (Alzheimer's Society, 2020a; Dementia UK, 2020a; Rare Dementia Support, 2020), with new discoveries continuing (NHS, 2019). There do seem to be some symptoms that are common to many types, such as short-term memory problems, word-finding difficulties and confusion (Alzheimer's Disease International, 2020). Others seem to be quite specific to certain types of dementia, such as hallucinations or visual-spatial difficulties (Dementia UK, 2020b). This is important to note because the term 'dementia' is typically used as an umbrella term for a wide range of conditions. This is because 'dementia' is considered in medical classification to be a 'syndrome', that is, 'a group of signs or symptoms whose appearance together usually indicates the presence of a particular disease or disorder' or 'a pattern or series of events, observed qualities, etc. characteristic of a particular problem or condition' (Chambers Dictionary [online], 2020).

In the UK, the term 'dementia' is typically used with reference to all of the specific types or diagnoses of progressive neurological impairment and this is as a result of key similarities they are considered to share. There are also conditions which can cause 'dementia-like' symptoms (and exacerbate symptoms in persons with dementia) but which are temporary or reversible, such as urinary-tract infections, the effects of poly-pharmacy, underactive thyroid and, particularly in older people, depression and delirium (Social Care Institute for Excellence, 2015a). The point to bear in mind is that 'dementia' is a term of convenience originating in, and perpetuated by, the clinical classification of symptoms associated with neurological disorders. There is more to say about the significance of the progressive aspect of dementia.

The symptoms of dementia, the impacts of progressive neurological conditions on individuals, get worse over time. This means that when faced with statements about 'people with dementia' it is vital to spot the danger of accepting blanket assumptions about everyone who has a diagnosis of dementia. In short, people have different types of dementia and their symptoms will be associated with their type of dementia. The severity of the symptoms people experience at any given time will also vary, and this relates to the degree of progression there has been in a person's neurological impairment associated with their type of dementia.

The primary outcome of beginning to question statements about 'dementia' is to learn that there are numerous types of specific conditions, as well as degrees of neurological impairment, which are commonly collapsed into the term. This should signal clearly that caution is required about presuming to know what 'dementia' any person might have and how this might be affecting them. Each person's experience of dementia is unique. A further outcome of adopting this critical approach is to pause and consider dementia claims made about people. Investigating just who is affected by dementia reveals that age is the biggest risk factor. That is, the older you get the more likely you are to develop dementia.

Now of course we already know that this claim (like all claims) about age and dementia should be examined carefully. In so doing, a reasonable conclusion to reach would be that claims about age and dementia tend typically to include all types of dementia as a single dependent variable. This is a further example of the way in which 'dementia' is used as a term of convenience, in this case, for analysis of prevalence in a population. People can develop types of dementia at a variety of points in adult life but most usually at age 65 years and above (NHS England, 2020). Though estimates vary, there are thought to be around 45,000 people in the UK aged under 65 years (Alzheimer's Society, 2020b) and around 800,000 people aged over 65 years with a type of dementia (Alzheimer's Research UK, 2020). This indicates that dementia is not simply something that happens in older age, although it is no doubt much more common in older age.

Therefore, 'people with dementia' does not connote a single homogenous group but, rather, includes people in middle adulthood as well as people in their older adult lives. The same approach can be taken to unpicking other variations which are otherwise potentially obscured in claims about 'people with dementia'. For example, two-thirds of people who have dementia are women (Social Care Institute for Excellence, 2020); dementia affects people regardless of ethnic background but is under-diagnosed in people from black and minority ethnic groups (which is another 'group' of 26,000 people to be unpicked (Social Care Institute for Excellence, 2020)) and within which important variations have been noted (e.g. Pham, Petersen, Walters *et al.*, 2018); and people with Down syndrome are at much heightened risk of developing Alzheimer's disease (YoungDementia UK, 2020). The only conclusion to come to from this brief questioning of the term 'people with dementia' is that there is tremendous diversity among the lives of those hidden behind the categorisation. It begs a fundamental question: how useful is the category 'people with dementia' to informing the care and support of the individuals it describes?

Creating a fair, productive and empowering space to think again about dementia care and support requires these kinds of questions to be asked. The only 'truth' that appears to be certain is that each person who has a diagnosis of dementia will experience their life lived with their dementia in a unique way. The relationship-centred approach described in this book accepts that persons with dementia may have impairments which impact on their capabilities in a range of ways, and that these impairments are variable and get more severe and significant over time. The biomedical reality of dementia is accepted but, crucially, post-diagnosis, this kind of knowledge does not help answer questions about how best to provide dementia care and support.

When persons with dementia are accepted and their lives valued as being as important as those without dementia, impairments are not presumed before they are encountered. Instead, impairments are anticipated as potential challenges to communication – the currency of care and support – but realised only if and when they impact on interaction, communication and decision-making. Difficulties with communication arising from the impairments associated with dementia might be expected but, if problems in communication occur, these are not simply viewed as the sole responsibility or 'fault' of the person with dementia.

As noted earlier, an important, relatively recent advance in thinking about dementia has been to begin to question whether certain difficulties experienced by persons with dementia are indeed 'symptoms' of a disease or syndrome. The advance has been in recognising that some of the behaviours these symptoms refer to may, in reality, originate in the influence that people *without* dementia have on persons with dementia. Let's look at each of the four 'symptoms' noted above. Jan Dewing's work on wandering (2006) has been inspirational in that she questioned whether or not wandering behaviour is a symptom of dementia. She concluded that the reasons that some persons with dementia walk about in care environments where they are receiving treatment or care can be the same reasons that anyone walks about in a care environment: boredom, seeking companionship, looking for somewhere else to go, pain relief, and being nosy. By extension, Dewing (2006) argues that it is the interpretation of care practitioners, with their legitimate concerns about safety and staffing levels, which can lead to such behaviour being viewed as problematic and, therefore, 'symptomised'.

Similarly, the belief that violence or challenging behaviour is a symptom of dementia has also been disputed (see e.g. Stokes, 2017). While some persons with dementia exhibit these kinds of behaviours, it has been argued that the causes can originate in care practitioners' attitudes and lack of awareness of the person's perspective, for example repeatedly ignoring persons with dementia, attempting to physically manoeuvre people in directions they do not want to go or speaking to people in off-hand or disrespectful ways. How would this make you feel? The conclusion suggested is that anyone, not just persons with dementia, would become animated or confrontational if provoked in these ways.

The idea that 'people with dementia tend to live in the past' refers to widely recognised symptoms of memory loss which accompany dementia. It is claimed that when someone has dementia their short-term memory is affected more adversely than their long-term memory. In response, many have championed reminiscence-based approaches within dementia care and support services (Gibson, 2004; Schweitzer and Bruce, 2008). In fact, the UK NHS has recently announced changes to some of its care environments to encourage reminiscence (NHS England, 2019) and there is growing popularity of care facilities in which facsimiles of 'historical' environments are presented as 'real' (Guardian, 2018). I agree that reminiscence, life story work (McKeown, Clarke, Ingleton *et al.*, 2010) and other narrative activities which encourage persons with dementia to tap into long-term memory – and experience a renewed sense of accomplishment, meaning and identity, and promote positive communication with others – have their place. However, if persons with dementia are predominantly offered opportunities to 'live in the past', then this, arguably, creates a situation whereby persons with dementia can do nothing but live a symptomised life, pickled in their own or some generic fictionalised past. If you are encouraged by others to live in the past, is it then fair to suggest it's your fault or the fault of your dementia?

Finally, in relation to the claim that people with dementia lack understanding, I draw on my postgraduate research undertaken some years ago (Reid, 1998). This focused on the ways that persons with dementia attending forms of day care described themselves, and how they were described by their respective family carers and care practitioners. In this research, I observed that care practitioners had, without intending to, developed a public lingua franca, their own vocabulary, for talking with persons with dementia about their dementia. For reasons which practitioners felt were justified, including not wanting to do harm, they would not use the term 'dementia' when service users asked them what was causing their difficulties. Instead, they would draw on discourses of normal ageing to explain to someone why they were becoming forgetful or confused (i.e. 'it's your age') (Reid, 1998).

To me, this had consequences for persons with dementia in terms of them being able to understand their situations and the reasons why they thought they were attending day-care services. Their lack of understanding about why they were in day-care services, revealed in interviews I conducted with them, and a focus on the interactions that persons with dementia had with care practitioners, suggested that attributing certain behaviour to symptoms of dementia makes invisible and discounts discussion of the influence and role practitioners can have in skewing people's understandings of their daily lives.

The dementia care and support practitioner, then, has a special role to play in the relationships he or she develops with persons with dementia and their families or supporters. The relationship-centred approach outlined in this book explores this role. In any episode of dementia care and support where a practitioner is present, there are typically three distinctive perspectives that they must acknowledge, identify and act on. These are now described below. The basic framework suggested is one that I adopt throughout the rest of the book to explore and develop a critical, relationship-centred approach in dementia care and support.

1. The person with dementia

The impairments caused by the progressive neurological syndrome of dementia on individuals are often simplified for convenience, that is, for the convenience of people without dementia. The vocabulary of 'dementia', 'people with dementia' and 'symptoms' conveys generalisations which have their place, but that place is not when seeking to understand the subjective experiences of individual human beings in order to offer support or care. In this respect, generalisations about 'people with dementia' are largely useless. Such simplifications are also out of step with the hugely progressive steps seen in the past 30 years to robustly assert and then seek understanding about the enduring humanity of people diagnosed with dementia. There is further discussion of those changes in thinking in Chapter 2.

One of the most important outcomes of this revolution in thinking about dementia is the shift towards presuming that persons with dementia are able to communicate and do possess knowledge, skills, ambitions, talents and opinions of tremendous value. Thus, in this relationship-centred approach, each person with dementia has to be encountered as a unique individual. The practitioner has to be able and willing to set aside or dump their accumulated 'dementia baggage' and adopt a critical perspective towards dementia knowledge. They must know that if they do not do this there is a real threat that it will contaminate their expectations of the person and adversely affect the communication relationships, and the care and support which follow.

It is the person, not their potentially contaminating dementia label, that is of interest, and the practitioner's role is to seek to understand what a person wants, feels and aspires to in any given situation. The legitimacy of a person's perspective is taken for granted and is not up for negotiation. The main work is to devote time and energy to the communication required with someone to understand their perspective, and to do this to the best of their 'conscience' (Reid, 1999).

2. The family member or supporter

Within any care or support encounter where a practitioner is involved there is also likely (but not always) to be a 'significant other' present, usually a family member but possibly a friend. It has already been noted that it is almost worthless attempting to generalise with regard to 'people with dementia' and so, I would argue, it is with 'carers' of persons with dementia – that is, apart from the conclusion that each family member and/or supporter will possess their own experience of life affected by dementia, one that is radically different from their loved one (though not always obviously so) whom they care for or support and who has a dementia diagnosis. They are all different, as people are all different.

Caring for or supporting a person with dementia occurs in a myriad of ways and for a myriad of reasons. Not everyone has chosen to be in the position of principal supporter, though many will view it as their duty or responsibility. Because people develop dementia at different ages, and of different types, and respond to associated impairments in unique ways, the particular perspective of the family member or supporter is not predictable. What is predictable is that they will have a unique perspective of their own, and this perspective is very likely to be of immense value to the practitioner. Their perspective is not only valuable in its own right but provides a source of knowledge about the person with dementia which, if possessed by the practitioner, can assist greatly in a rounded, historical appreciation of the person.

Acknowledging this expertise also sends a clear message to the family member or supporter that they are vitally important to the care and support provided by others, now and in the future, and this can be absolutely crucial in determining the quality of the care and support that a person is offered. It is with these insights in mind that this relationship-centred approach requires that practitioners also acknowledge, respect and seek to understand the perspective of the family member or supporter. More ideas about this role, its importance and how such expertise can be obtained and put into practice are outlined in Chapter 3. However, in the approach I am suggesting, it is important for practitioners to accept that they must be orientated towards offering care and support to both the person with dementia *and* their family member or supporter. This leaves one further perspective for the practitioner to appreciate.

3. The dementia care practitioner

In many discussions of dementia care and support it is frequently the case that the care practitioner's role is taken as given. Those working with persons with dementia are automatically expected to have the necessary skills and abilities, or some training is provided which usually distils to a list of things to learn about 'dementia'. There is rarely, if ever, a recommendation to seek to learn from persons with dementia and their families or supporters. Similarly, there is rarely mention of the expertise which practitioners have already learned or might be learned from collective discussion within teams. Also, there is usually no discussion of the impact on practitioners of working closely with persons with dementia and their families, and about what support they might require.

In reality, a lot of the time, the dementia practitioner is considered virtually irrelevant to discussions of care and support. They are given prescribed dementia information or expected to unpack obscure policy goals, such as making your practice 'dementia friendly', which they are expected to understand and enact. The general expectation with this kind of engagement with practitioners is that this 'top-down' knowledge transfer will lead to improved outcomes for persons with dementia. Until individuals or a workforce are required for the purpose of apportioning blame for care not delivered to the standards over-promised by policy, the practitioner is virtually invisible. In contrast to this, in a relationship-centred approach to dementia care, the practitioner is valued in the same ways it is suggested they value the person with dementia and family members or supporters. In order for practitioners to engage in the tasks of authentic communication, care and support of persons with dementia and their families or supporters, they themselves require serious consideration as skilled, knowledgeable workers, and as human beings. Like persons with dementia in the past, dementia practitioners have been ignored, institutionalised, marginalised and often blamed for the problems of dementia.

Of course, this is not always the case. There have been incidents of incompetence and abuse perpetrated by practitioners as well as, collectively, by health care organisations and regulatory bodies, and these are condemned (e.g. Parliamentary and Health Service Ombudsman, 2011; The Francis Report, 2013; Cooper, Marston, Barber *et al.*, 2018). What is written here does not in any way exonerate or excuse such behaviour. At the same time, however, I argue there is a problem with a situation where practitioners who support and care for persons with dementia are undervalued and under-supported and simply expected to engage in the highly skilled and complex work of dementia care and support, viewed as possessing unlimited reserves, little critical facility and no expert knowledge of their own.

This book is not aimed directly at employers and managers of dementia care and support services, at members of associated governance bodies or at politicians. Yet, it should be obvious that high-quality dementia care, whether organised in a relationship-centred way or not, requires management which values appropriately the practitioner's role – that is, management which understands practitioners' needs, and, in response, supplies the necessary resources to facilitate the sustainable delivery of high-quality dementia care and support. One of the significant limitations of Kitwood's (1997b, p.17) ideas about dementia care is the implication that the existence of a 'malignant social-psychology' (or poor culture of care) can be addressed by adjustments in the behaviours and attitudes of practitioners in that setting, as if organisational and institutional factors play no part. The organisational context is latent but fundamental to what can be achieved and maintains its invisibility in many discussions of dementia care. In Chapter 6, suggestions are made about how practitioners can connect with management (and vice versa) within organisations to create feedback loops to support excellence in dementia care and support.

The relationship-centred approach outlined here is one which views the practitioner as pivotal, someone capable of negotiating the uncertain every day with persons with dementia, their families or supporters but also of initiating action, doing, leading the episode of care or support insofar as they take responsibility to acknowledge and then seek to access and utilise the uniquely valuable expertise of those they support or care for. Mindful of their own limitations, prejudices and fears, the relationship-centred dementia care practitioner *learns* what to do from the education available to them from persons with dementia, their families and supporters. Education is the central organising principle of this approach to relationship-centred care and this is now explained in the final part of this chapter.

4. Introducing an educational perspective to dementia care and support

I have contributed to the development of ideas about relationship-centred dementia care elsewhere (Nolan, Ryan, Enderby *et al.*, 2002; Ryan, Nolan, Reid *et al.*, 2008). I develop some of these ideas, in particular the analytical value of the Senses Framework (Ryan, Nolan, Reid *et al.*, 2008), by looking differently at the nature of interactions between persons with dementia, family members or supporters and practitioners in episodes of care. Specifically, the version of relationship-centred care I outline examines, to some degree, power relations; identifies who has designated responsibility for interaction and action in care encounters; and refers to the practical challenges facing practitioners of achieving and maintaining familiarity with persons with dementia, their family members and supporters.

The Senses Framework remains an excellent route by which to conceptualise and then examine the outcomes of care and support for persons with dementia, family members and dementia care practitioners (Ryan, Nolan, Enderby *et al.*, 2004; Ryan, Nolan, Reid *et al.*, 2008; see also Tresolini and the Pew-Fetzer Task Force, 1994). Nothing in the past 20 years has led me to change my view that the most important focus for understanding what actually goes on and what is possible in dementia care is communication, interaction and action, involving the practitioner, person with dementia and family member or supporter. This is distinct from ideas about personhood and what became known as person-centred care, which neither instinctively nor by revision prompted an equality of gaze towards the three main participants in care and support.

My critical, relationship-centred approach begins with the simple premise that all members of the care and support 'triad' (Reid, 1997) are significant and of significant concern. It does not begin with a concern to understand and protect the human rights of persons with dementia (Cahill, 2018), a concern which, sadly, echoes the historical battle to assert the continuing humanity of persons with dementia (Woods, 1989). Neither does it seek to do justice to the great potential understanding offered by a full exploration of a social model of dementia (Gilliard, Means, Beattie *et al.*, 2005) or of what citizenship means when a person has dementia (Bartlett, 2014). Nor does it seek to examine how the recovery model of dementia offers ways of promoting greater empowerment in care and support services (Gavan, 2011). All of these endeavours have tremendous potential value. Instead, the triad – the person with dementia, the family member or supporter and the care practitioner – comprises a basic unit of analysis, and all of the concerns noted above could be explored by its use.

Where I would like to develop a new way of conceptualising relationship-centred dementia care is to argue that a crucial feature of these relationships is their educational function and potential. In this view, practitioners, persons with dementia and family members or supporters are engaged in learning and teaching. If each participant in the three-way relationship is positioned as being in possession of unique expert knowledge, thus moving away from the language of 'needs' or the relativistic 'senses of' – which are always vulnerable to subjective quantification – there is a decisive shift towards equality of consideration.

Where this chimes with me is in terms of my experiences of learning from persons with dementia, a significant influence on how I have come to my view of dementia care and dementia education. I have already mentioned Harry's influence (Reid, 1996). This was, I realised retrospectively, a significant epiphany. A rather mechanical exploration of the effectiveness of data collection methods was eclipsed by the realisation that I was being taught something I didn't know by a person with dementia. Further research I helped conduct confirmed that persons with dementia were 'discerning' and had individual opinions about the kind of support they wanted, if they were asked to share these (Reid, Ryan and Enderby, 2001). Later, I consulted persons with dementia, as well as family members and supporters and practitioners, about what to teach on a dementia course (Reid and Witherspoon, 2008), and the content of a dementia information booklet distributed at NHS memory clinics (Reid, Warnes and Low, 2014). I also supported persons with dementia to teach undergraduate and postgraduate students.

I have also coordinated annual dementia creative arts exhibitions in South Yorkshire (Reid, 2014) and in Michigan (USA) with John Wood, an artist who has dementia (Wood, Reid and Marks, 2016; Wood, 2020). John has patiently taught me a lot about how to improve exhibitions but, most importantly, it is in his work teaching people about life lived with dementia by putting into the public domain his original artwork that has had the greatest impact. In fact, all persons with dementia who contribute to the exhibitions contribute to public knowledge about dementia as well as to our cultural life (Basting, 2018).

My view is that when persons with dementia are positioned as educators, with unique expertise to convey, two things happen. First, that person has available to them a source of self-esteem which may have been eroded or endangered since their diagnosis. Second, those working with persons with dementia experience a shift in their expectations towards the person, from anticipating a care recipient or partner in care to meeting an expert, knowledgeable and of equal status in discussions. It is these expectations which practitioners have of persons with dementia that are particularly crucial to isolate and explore.

My view, which is influenced strongly by ideas about social identity and its maintenance (Mead, 1934; Sabat and Harrè, 1992; Golander and Raz, 1996; Vittoria, 1998; Sabat, 2001), is that practitioners are uniquely placed to offer persons with dementia opportunities for continuation of social identity and, crucially, opportunities for new sources of identity and self-esteem. At the same time, and through the same processes, dementia care practitioners have new opportunities for enhanced self-esteem, self-development and job satisfaction.

A clear statement about dementia expertise can be made in approaching dementia care and support in this way. It is not the preserve of academics or self-appointed dementia 'gurus': dementia expertise is learned through personal experience by those most closely affected and only conveyed when opportunities are provided for this to be heard and acted on. At its core, a critical, relationship-centred dementia care approach is a mutually educative enterprise. Once one considers persons with dementia and family members and supporters to be experts in their own experiences it is only logical to begin to ask questions about what range of opportunities people have to share their experiences, be heard and understood, and about what it is they are communicating and what action should come next. This is the domain and responsibility of the dementia care and support practitioner. In Chapter 2, the focus is firmly on how practitioners can learn from persons with dementia.

■ CHAPTER 2 ■

Learning from Persons with dementia

Once you adopt an educational perspective towards the care and support of persons with dementia there is liberation from the narrow thinking associated with dealing with human beings as medical labels. The uncritical adoption of a biomedical perspective encourages confirmatory approaches, whereby the person without dementia views and judges the person with dementia primarily in terms of looking for evidence of symptoms or attributing what a person says or does to their dementia. It is a dehumanising gaze, which originates in the person without dementia. The good news is that by reflecting critically on the ways we without dementia frame the person with dementia it is possible to question our dementia knowledge and then begin to develop fairer and exciting new approaches which, in turn, can have transformative effects for persons with dementia.

In this chapter, the critical, relationship-centred approach that I advocate is explored by focusing on the first of the three main perspectives which dementia care practitioners must value: that of persons with dementia. Some context is offered for what nowadays is, and should be, accepted wisdom: that each person with dementia is the expert when it comes to their own experiences.

It has taken some time to advance to this point, and with no little struggle. Even so, this position feels precarious, fragile, unset and is accepted more readily for some than it is for others. Following this discussion, examples are provided from my research and interactions with persons with dementia to give a flavour of what can be learned – the sorts of insights and knowledge from which I and others have benefited hugely.

Setting the scene

Some persons with dementia are now setting the agenda for action, policy, understanding and support provided in their name. For examples of this, you need go no further than examining the work of the Dementia Engagement and Empowerment Project (DEEP), from the UK Network of Dementia Voices (Dementia Engagement and Empowerment Project, 2020a), which started in 2011 as a one-year project to map 'involvement groups' in the UK. DEEP's broader mission is now to 'engage and empower people living with dementia to influence attitudes, services and policies that affect their lives'. DEEP organises groups across the UK and is independent; its groups are diverse and it operates on a 'rights-based approach' whereby groups of persons with dementia are encouraged to identify and speak out about the issues that are important to them. One of their projects is *Dementia Enquirers* (Dementia Engagement and Empowerment Project, 2020b), which aims to develop 'a new approach to research, or "enquiry", that is led and controlled by people with dementia'. It has individuals active within it who bestride multiple other organisations, both national and international, pressing for positive change, informed by their own and others' expertise and experiences.

In the UK, there are other organisations (e.g. Innovations in Dementia, 2020) that are configured to empower persons with dementia. One notable project is the *Dementia Diaries* (2020) initiative, whereby persons with dementia record and then publish online news of their daily lives. In these and other examples there is undeniable evidence of the over-used but nonetheless powerful demand for self-advocacy, 'Nothing about us without us'. These communities of persons with dementia, facilitated by allies, also enhance public 'awareness' of dementia or public education about dementia, as do published autobiographical accounts such as those by Kate Swaffer (2016) and Wendy Mitchell (2018).

These advances have not occurred by chance but have been 30 years in the making. In offering some historical context for how in the present day we must now approach persons with dementia as experts, there is a danger of crediting only those who reported what they discovered to be unexpected and 'new'. This danger is apparent in a number of current thorny discussions in society, ranging from the rightful ownership and guardianship of artefacts on display in British museums (Museums Association, 2019) to the febrile, worldwide debate sparked in 2020 about the acceptability of statues of historical figures continuing to occupy public spaces in light of urgent questions which followed the murder of George Floyd on 25 May in Minnesota, USA, and the Black Lives Matter protests (Guardian, 2020a). Changing attitudes to cultural property and statues are discussions about historical acts of appropriation, about taking something that was someone else's, silencing 'other' people in history and, simultaneously, gaining from those acts.

In dementia, this issue of appropriation has been pointed to by Page and Fletcher (2006; see also O'Brien, 1996; Maurer, Volk and Gerbaldo, 1997) who write about the life of Auguste Durat, the woman whose condition was described by the rather better known Alois Alzheimer and colleagues (see Stelzmann, Schnitzlein and Murtagh, 1995). By bringing out of the shadows the woman whose life is at the very centre of scientific dementia knowledge, the authors raise vital questions about the way we approach and value dementia expertise and knowledge. Over the years, I have reminded myself and sought to convince others of the necessity of exploring what Post's ideas about 'an epistemology of humility' (Post, 2001, p.18) in dementia might mean for decisions we make about whose voices are heard and whose agendas are followed.

'Out of the shadows' is a metaphor used frequently in discussions of dementia (e.g. Alzheimer's Society, 2008; Irish Times, 2014; Seattle Times, 2018). One argument is that if one accepts that appropriation has occurred in dementia, the next steps include returning the 'cultural property' to those who rightfully own it, for the old 'statues' to be removed elsewhere or replaced. What might this mean for dementia knowledge and who history credits for advances in thinking? Would there be resistance? In some ways, the change is already occurring. When universities and academics are superseded by self-organising groups of persons with dementia advocating on their own behalf, speaking for themselves, then the 'seats of knowledge' and of power have moved. The 'University of Dementia', an idea I helped develop (Wood, Reid and Marks, 2016), would see persons with dementia in key teaching roles (see Chapter 8).

Following the same rationale, family members and supporters, as well as dementia care and support practitioners, would all have key teaching roles. Then, with people affected by dementia at the centre of dementia education, civil rights, policy and public education, would it be time to seek 'reparations' for those persons with dementia who were shut away, not listened to, marginalised from society from the UK County Asylums Act of 1808 (The National Archives, 2020) onwards?

With all of this in mind it is, with regret, not possible to name all of the persons with dementia who helped advance our thinking to where we are today. This is for a number of reasons but primary among them is the fact that in published academic research, one of the key sites for evidence of changes in thinking, the names of persons with dementia have been changed. This is normal practice in all academic research and is justifiable on the basis that individuals have a right to anonymity which is offered 'as standard' during the process of seeking informed consent to participate. However, what this means is that it is impossible to attribute/distribute credit fairly to those who have precipitated a revolution in our understanding of persons with dementia. Persons with dementia were always there but, as Bev Graham puts it, 'nobody's actually bothered to ask them' (Sheffield Health and Social Care NHS Foundation Trust and the Alzheimer's Society Sheffield, 2013).

Instead, and it is not their fault, it is the authors of academic studies in which persons with dementia provide the basis of new understandings who have, generally speaking, become associated with the expertise. It is perhaps a bitter irony that many of those whose voices and experiences have taught us to listen to persons with dementia shall remain unknown. With this caveat, and apology, what follows is my brief account of some key moments in the emergence of a growing realisation that persons with dementia have been ignored and marginalised.

Starting away from academic research, Robert Davis (1989), Diana Friel McGowin (1993) and Larry Rose (1996) all wrote and published autobiographical accounts which indicated that some could teach us directly about their lives lived with dementia, and the ripple effects on families and occupations. In each book, the author tells of how they first noted the changes that indicated something had changed, that something was wrong, and their various attempts to hide these from loved ones. They also report how diagnoses were sought and how this news was given and received.

Reporting from within the context of real lives, Robert, Diana and Larry offer insights from the examples of their daily lives. If you read these accounts it is interesting to note the similar, diary-like, quality as each person provides a chronology of before, during and after diagnosis. Interestingly, Larry Rose states he was inspired to write his book after reading Diana Friel McGowin's book (Rose, 1996).

The emergence of these rich and poignant accounts occurred at around the same time that Donna Cohen (1991) argued it was time for a better understanding of the subjective experiences of persons with dementia. A few years earlier, she and a colleague (Cohen and Eisdorfer, 1986) published a book entitled *The Loss of Self*, in which they drew on excerpts from their consultations with persons with dementia to demonstrate that such people had varying degrees of awareness of the sorts of changes that were occurring to them. Fundamentally, Cohen and Eisdorfer (1986) demonstrated the continuing potential of communication when at the time, elsewhere, the dominant belief appeared to be that persons with dementia should be considered to be 'empty shells' or 'coping with a living death' (Woods, 1989). Language guides, informed by persons with dementia, are now available to help ensure that more acceptable terminology is used (e.g. Dementia Engagement and Empowerment Project, 2014; Alzheimer's Society, 2018; Dementia Australia, 2020). The usage of dementia language provides evidence of how thinking has changed over time.

Back in the late 1980s and early 1990s, as someone who became interested in what persons with dementia had to say, I found it very powerful to encounter work such as that undertaken with care home residents by the writer and poet John Killick (1994). The 'poems' that Killick constructed from the words of individual residents with whom he communicated spoke to me of locked-away, forgotten and confused people, trying to make the best sense they could of their everyday lives. At the time, momentum was beginning to grow for a reappraisal of assumptions about persons with dementia, a reappraisal that continues to this day.

Different insights began to be added together and a community of interest developed. Tom Kitwood (1989, 1990, 1993a, 1993b, 1997a, 1997b) and Kathleen Bredin (Kitwood and Bredin, 1992) developed and shared revolutionary ideas about the enduring psychological lives of those with dementia, challenging directly the dominance and adequacy of biomedical approaches to dementia.

Rightly, in my view, Kitwood's work is often cited as being crucial in creating new space/s to think about dementia. For me, the most valuable result of his industrious and determined period of writing was to shift attention from the fixation with organic brain disease towards consideration of the interaction between those without dementia and their impact on those with dementia. Kitwood did not argue for autonomy or self-advocacy; his view was that 'people with dementia' in general should be considered, to one degree or another, dependent on the care of others (Kitwood, 1997a). In the light of the dementia activist movements of today this now seems a simplistic assumption. However, by arguing convincingly that a person with dementia retained psychological needs, a psychological self, Kitwood and Bredin opened a door that did not exist previously to discussion and consideration of how others, those without dementia – in particular, dementia care practitioners – could, through their attitudes, behaviour and actions, exact a positive (or negative) impact on persons with dementia. For Kitwood, this impact was highly significant in that it could be equated with positive or negative effects on a person's psychological resources that are available to help them cope with their life with dementia.

Kitwood spent a lot of time with persons with dementia to gain the insights which informed his thinking. He had his own subjectivity to deal with, too. His extended and wide-ranging ideas about 'personhood' are frequently couched in ways which tend to suggest a Christian faith (Kitwood, 1997a) and his earlier writings are presented in a format which demonstrated the fight he had on to convince his academic peers of his arguments, such as in the use of equations to seek to 'prove' the enduring humanity of people with dementia (Kitwood, 1990). Looking back, this reveals something of the struggle to change people's minds about dementia, to prompt people to think again. Elsewhere, others called for disciplines not typically associated with the study of dementia to get involved and contribute their energy and perspectives to re-imagining approaches to care and support (Lyman, 1989).

Some who responded to the prevailing zeitgeist included sociologists such as Sabat and Harrè (1992), Golander and Raz (1996) and Vittoria (1998). These academics spoke with persons with dementia, examined and thought about what they said and raised questions about what this indicated about their enduring yet vulnerable social identities. Crucially, these studies linked what persons with dementia said with how this information was valued by dementia care practitioners. In Vittoria's (1998) research, the implication was clear: that practitioners could seek actively to 'preserve' a person's social identity if they took the trouble to learn about a person and their life, value it and then offer opportunities for the continuation of the social roles individuals valued themselves.

A further notable contributor in the early challenge to the dominance of biomedical ideas about dementia, and their erasing effects, was the collective endeavours of Dementia Advocacy and Support Network International (DASNI). DASNI was, so far as I am aware, the first online community and activist group where a large proportion of members were persons with dementia. Their website no longer exists (see Dementia Alliance International, 2017), but in the 1990s it was a huge privilege to have permission to read and contribute to this community of people affected by dementia. From the early 1990s onwards, pioneers such as Carole Mullikan and Tracy Mobley (Mobley, 2007), across North America and further afield, began communicating online with others affected by dementia via mailing list software, offering advice, sharing experiences and support and keeping in touch with one another. This online community included a core of individuals who made representations to local, state and national government in the United States, on behalf of persons with dementia.

This kind of online community continues today in other, more mature forms, such as Dementia Alliance International, which is exclusively for the use of people diagnosed with dementia. These online forms of peer support and activism are also easy to find on generic social media platforms where persons with dementia have, undoubtedly, much greater access to each other, and ability to connect with those without dementia – to have a voice – than at any other time in history.

This whistle-stop tour of some key moments in changes to thinking about dementia is not intended to be definitive. In fact, it would be very useful if someone were to present a comprehensive historical account to enlighten new and old about how persons with dementia contributed to new thinking to provide a counter-weight and complement to the history of academic publications. At this point, it is sufficient to state that many persons with dementia have played and continue to play their part in helping those of us without dementia – along with persons with dementia – understand what it is like for them to live with their dementia. It is simply that we do not know who to thank. There are also others to thank, such as persons with dementia who agreed to donate their brains to medical research after death, so that scientists and, by extension, wider society might understand better the causes of the syndrome and provide the raw material for potential interventions to alleviate and, one day, develop treatments for dementia.

I labour this point deliberately because it begs two relevant, related but rarely asked questions. I invite you now to ask yourself these questions:

- What have I learned from persons with dementia?

- Have I given credit to those persons with dementia for what they have taught me?

The questions can be posed at a number of levels, not just the personal, though that is a good starting point. For example, have you learned anything about the subtleties of interpersonal communication and how to facilitate this, about the value of humour or the significance of personal biography to communication and understanding behaviour? Have you learned new things about local history, about the ways that places and people's roles have changed over time? Have you learned things about what's important in life, about what really matters?

And, shifting levels, dementia policy is being informed by persons with dementia at local and national levels, for example in contributions made to national dementia strategies. We learn from dementia knowledge produced by the academic community engaging with persons with dementia. This is found in publications which range from reporting the social-psychological impact of dementia on people to those reporting clinical findings of neurological and pathological research.

In each instance, it is persons with dementia who provide the basis for learning and I believe that these people fail to receive the recognition they deserve for the expertise that, one way or another, they have shared and continue to share. If you were not able to answer the questions above, I set you a personal challenge. Start to look for and identify the ways that persons with dementia offer you learning, both on an individual level – the people you meet and with whom you interact – and collectively, through their contribution to other forms of dementia knowledge that you consume. By beginning to acknowledge that relationships with persons with dementia are two-way streets, where knowledge, expertise, commitment, humour and personality are exchanged by both parties, we begin a meaningful process of maintaining value in that person or revaluing that person, with all that follows on from that position.

There are, therefore, a variety of rich resources available now to learn from persons with dementia about their experiences. There are two warnings that I would give about this kind of learning and this refers particularly to research reported in academic journals. The first is an extension of a point made in Chapter 1, that claims about 'people with dementia' are largely useless. The vast majority of studies in which opinion is sought from persons with dementia are, necessarily, studies involving very few numbers. It is very important to remain aware of the limitation this places on generalisation. Most academics worth their salt will highlight this limitation but not all are as attentive. Given that possession of a dementia diagnosis is the only guaranteed similarity between those participating in studies – and that the level and type of impairment varies – the claims that can be made about people with dementia are highly circumspect. Even when diligent authors highlight the limits to generalisation, there often remains a tendency to make claims about 'people with dementia'. I highlight my own previous research to be among this group (e.g. Reid, Ryan and Enderby, 2001) rather than name others here. Look out for this tendency in the research you read. Much more thought and discussion is required about the relevance of dementia research to all persons with dementia.

Second, caution is also required about equating what academic research focuses on – in terms of just what it is that persons with dementia are asked to offer their perspectives on, i.e. the subject – with what persons with dementia themselves view as most pressing or significant in their lives. This is a point that I elaborate on towards the end of this chapter in relation to other research I have conducted. Academic research is largely based on academics applying for grants from a range of organisations to fund their work. There are requirements in place within many funding organisations for academics to demonstrate that they have consulted with 'stakeholders' in the design of their studies (National Institute for Health Research Involve, 2020), and this includes persons with dementia. At a university level, there is a further driver to involve stakeholders such as persons with dementia, in order that they can write up impact case studies identifying the benefits of their research, as part of the Research Excellence Framework (2014) cycle, which, in turn, influence decisions made about how much central government funding for research is allocated to each higher education institution (i.e. university, research centre) (Research England, 2020).

While these requirements and mechanisms to encourage the involvement of persons with dementia are undeniably positive, it should also be clear that the academic/s involved play the lead role in deciding what the focus of the research should be. It is with some mystification that I have read studies exploring the significance of exercise or the importance of companion animals or of fresh air to persons with dementia. I find myself removing the 'with dementia' from the study title or conclusions and thinking, 'No shit, Sherlock!' It does make me wonder whether this kind of research actually perpetuates the separation of persons with dementia from society rather than promotes acceptance and inclusion.

The sort of research noted above seems at one level to represent an ongoing and extended re-evaluation of arguments that persons with dementia are people. In my view, the academic dementia 'industry' needs to be subject to greater scrutiny to ensure it is not simply creating work for itself. Do we really need to check, human characteristic by human characteristic, as if seeking to create and be persuaded by some vast person-shaped collage, that persons with dementia remain human beings? Do you still need proof?

I do not wish to suggest that any specific academic intends to do this but the net result of viewing such studies is to ask: whose idea was it to focus on this particular subject and why? In summary, this point is again one about ownership, expertise and the generation of knowledge. It seems to me that if academic researchers can account for their focus by demonstrating it originates in agendas set by persons with dementia then this research is likely to be of more value to persons with dementia.

Dementia care and support practitioners are consumers of dementia knowledge and expertise. What has been outlined so far in this chapter includes resources to access to enhance your knowledge and a suggestion that you ask some critical questions about it. Remember, these critical questions are not for the purpose of discounting the value of these resources – far from it. Instead, they are to encourage you to be clear about the pros and cons of what it is you are learning, the insights and the limitations. Each dementia care practitioner will have his or her own 'learning journey', if you like, and this will include insights gained from their own personal interactions. This strand of learning is elaborated on in Chapter 4, which focuses on the practitioner's experiences of dementia.

For now, attention turns to sharing some of my learning from persons with dementia. The purpose here is to bring to life this personal process of learning by using examples from my own research and other interactions. Taking the advice I gave above, I try to identify what I learned, give credit to those I learned from (where this is permissible) and explain why certain individuals were prompted to talk about the topics they discuss.

My learning from persons with dementia

As the main aim of this chapter is to explore the value of learning from persons with dementia, I have decided to focus on a chronology of learning episodes. I summarise the main points from this learning at the end and I emphasise the personal nature of this learning. A chronology of main learning from persons with dementia starts with Harry, as noted in the Preface. Harry's description of his work as a printer for Hansard, and his use of the word 'clitch', had me scurrying to my dictionary and the realisation, in a word, that this man with dementia had taught me something. In what follows, I outline four episodes in which I identify significant learning. The first was research undertaken with persons with dementia attending day-care services in Scotland. The second episode was a focus group meeting with members of a peer support group of persons with dementia in South Yorkshire. This is followed by an account of my learning which comes from my ongoing association with John Wood, a US-based artist and teacher. Finally, I refer to learning inspired by Colin Ward.

Persons with dementia attending day-care services

This postgraduate research study was motivated by my own desire to understand more about the ways persons with dementia describe themselves, when given the opportunity, and how these descriptions compared with descriptions of the people concerned which were obtained from their family members and from dementia care practitioners. Focusing on the interviews I conducted with day-care attenders, I made a decision to get to know possible interviewees by spending time in the day-care settings so that I could develop rapport, get a sense of who I should and should not ask to take part in a conversational interview, and to begin a process of asking selected individuals whether or not they would like to take part.

I called this the 'familiarity phase', and my decision to do so was based on insights I had gained while undertaking my previous research with Harry and others and an appreciation of process consent (Usher and Arthur, 1998) – a way of approaching individuals to participate which gave them multiple opportunities to ask questions or seek clarification about my motives and the research that I was undertaking. Clearly, one way of viewing what I was doing was that I was seeking to replicate for myself an appreciation of the individuals in the settings which the dementia care practitioners developed in the course of their everyday work.

There are a couple of important points to note about how I explained what I was doing to persons with dementia in the settings. First, unless someone told me that they had a dementia diagnosis, I did not mention it. To these people, and it was the majority, I explained that I was interested in 'people like you who come to places like this', specifying the name of the place if it had an obvious name. Second, I deliberately structured the interviews so that (more or less) an equal amount of time was spent asking the person about their life in 'the past', 'the present' and their thoughts about 'the future'. At the time, I felt that studies had not paid attention to 'allowing' persons with dementia to speak about their 'presents' and their 'futures'.

These interviews, typically for an hour, varied considerably. Below, I present a few of the key themes that I felt were justified from the interviews. However, the focus is primarily on what these individuals said.

IDEAS ABOUT THE PRESENT, THE HERE AND NOW OF EVERYDAY LIFE AND THE FUTURE

Cliff knew he had a diagnosis of Alzheimer's disease, and when I spoke with him about his views on 'the present' he provided interesting points about the benefits of people like him being supported by care and support practitioners. Cliff attended a men-only 'day-care' service located in a volunteer's house, which ran once or twice a week.

> I expect as this group, the group cannae dae enough for any of us. Because, people who gi's up their privacy in their house is a great thing. And if you can go you meet different people. People who you've seen in the street and you'll say, 'Do you want to speak about this?' And you meet in a refuge… You've got another life there and you'll never starve, you'll never do without, they'll help you. [Pause] But as I say I would rather…with a stranger than a close relative. It's maybe funny but to me it's 'no'. The way I look at it is, at least what the people I've met, some I would dedicate myself to – say 'Right! That's it. You look after me.' And I think they look after you better than your own relations. [Pause] 'Cause, all they [relations] worry about I think is about how much money I'm going to leave.

I wasn't sure if Susan knew she had a diagnosis of dementia. I had been told she did, but I didn't bring it up. Like Cliff, Susan's view of the present also included the perceived benefits of having support. I was interested by the sort of attitudes she had towards everyday life and to the future. Susan attended a similar type of service to Cliff, located in another volunteer's home.

> Well, you're no sittin' looking out the window, for once. And sometimes we go away around to where they sell the plants and things… And we do different things when the weather's better, you know. But it's, you look forward to Tuesday and er, Friday… It's a great life. I mean thank to God I'm still living and that so, you just live as long as you can, hey?… Just keepin' yourself happy, I mean no bein' crabbit or anything like that, you know. I like to make everything alright. There are some people, I mean, who'll no talk to you, to cut their nose off, you know, and things like that.

No, I wouldnae do that. It's not so bad, I mean you're no havin' to work. You get your work done for you – the home help or things like that – it's good!

Again, I didn't know if Arthur knew he had a dementia diagnosis. He also had his views about the future and, when he paused, I asked him if he was a religious man.

Well, the future itself seems a long way off. But it's not as long off as you think it is. [Starts to cry] I've heard the second coming's beat for years. Still hasn't yet. Be it daylight or flashes. Though that happens it's not to say the world is finished. It still goes on. [Pause] Well, I wouldnae say I was a religious man. Religion doesnae mean anything to me. It's actually the spiritual welfare that's in the country or in the – that's what I'm saying. The spirit of men is alright but you must have good thought in your heart. That's the big, big problem. You look at your map, you look at your sun. It never moves. You know that? It's the Earth that moves – I learnt it at school – around the sun, 24 hours. The weather and that – that's all controlled by the maker Himself. And we can't do anythin' about it at all.

These three excerpts from Cliff, Susan and Arthur made me realise the significance the person without dementia (me) has in influencing the kinds of things that persons with dementia speak about, or show themselves to be interested in or are capable of commenting on. Being 'offered' the opportunity to speak about their sense of the present and their views about the future, persons with dementia spoke about them.

Focus group meeting with members of a peer support group of persons with dementia

A group of people attending a dementia peer support group agreed to speak with me when I started to write this book some years ago. I asked the group for any advice that they would like to give dementia care and support practitioners. The response was lengthy, and only a short section of this is reproduced below:

Treat you as an individual. (Female 1)

Be patient. (Male 1)

Sometimes they don't look at you, they talk over you. Instead of looking at you. (Female 1)

A lot of them, at our place for argument's sake, they're bedridden. Sit in their chairs all day, they can't talk and they sit and cry. And they cry for a reason. If you were 90 years old and in there, they shout at them: 'For goodness sake stop crying! What are you crying for?! Don't know? Well, stop it then!' That's wrong, isn't it? That woman's crying for a reason. I don't know why she's crying. Probably doesn't know herself. And I hate that when they shout at them. At toilet and things: 'Bloomin' heck! You going to the toilet again?! Come on then! But make sure you do something!' Well, I mean, when you're 90 years old you don't expect that type of treatment, do you? But I do hate to hear him when they shout at them for cryin' over doing something. 'For goodness sake! Get up – I've told you it's lunch time!' You know, it's not very nice. Well I think it's with me living there, when we've got visitors, everything's nice and lovely: 'Oh come on love,' you know. 'Your daughter's here, want a cup of tea?' I mean to be fair, some of the carers are wonderful, I mean I'm only talking about one or two who are a bit sharp and I think one day that could be happening to me, that. (Male 1)

I've not come across that one. My husband's in a care home but I've never come across that. It may exist, I don't know. I have never seen anything like that. (Female 1)

I mean there only has to be one bad egg in the basket doesn't there? (Male 1)

I think anybody there, they should make the person feel relaxed because if they get stressed up they have even more difficulties with the deficiencies, with memory and things. Stress, you know, makes things worse. If they can, when they're interviewing you, if they can create a sort of relaxed atmosphere, it's much better and you can sort of express yourself much better. (Male 2)

I say that you've got the person who's coming in and saying to the patient, like me, 'This is Mrs so-and-so and she's got difficulties.' But, you've got to be kind. You've got to think, you've got to try and think what they're thinking of. It's no good saying: 'Oh, come on, hurry up! Can you work a little bit quicker?' You can't do that. You've got to say: 'Let's take our time' and we'll go away. It's the worst thing out, listening to anybody who's like us, who's got dementia. Because it's not fair. We are ordinary people and even I can get angry. I get angry with myself at home – I say, 'You silly old moo!' But, this is it, you've got to be very careful and you've got to be kind, in a certain way... And I think that's where you can get the, you know, you don't want to be high up, you don't want to be too low. You've to be in the middle, haven't you? And I think that's what they've got to try and do with people. (Female 2)

I think it should be a carer's nature though, some women and men are nice and kind and some can be a bit angry, can't they? (Male 2)

There's qualifications but you can simply be nice to people, can't you? (Male 1)

One thing is patience. (Male 3)

That's about it, you've hit the jackpot! (Male 2)

Really you just want simple kindness. (Male 3)

Simple kindness and love. To feel that they look after you, not snapping your head off and saying to women, you know, 'What are you crying for?! Come on, bed!' (Male 3)

To want to do the job. (Male 2)

They have to treat you with respect. (Male 3)

And don't talk down to you. (Male 2)

Being proactive. (Male 3)

The insights provided by this group of persons with dementia identify some worrying behaviours among some dementia care and support practitioners. Overall, however, these people knew what qualities of care and support they liked because they had personal experience of how that feels.

John Wood, a US-based artist and teacher

I have worked with John Wood for a number of years now. He and I were introduced when he contacted me from Grosse Point, Michigan, asking to take part in the South Yorkshire Dementia Creative Arts Exhibition. He has contributed several times since and has coordinated sister exhibitions in the United States, putting on show artwork created by people affected by dementia from South Yorkshire, among other endeavours (see e.g. National Dementia Action Alliance, 2019; Wood, 2020). I asked John, with his wife Carol, to explain a little of what he thinks dementia care and support practitioners can learn from artwork created by persons with dementia:

> Well I think that when the people within the constellation of the diagnosis, including the person with dementia, their family and care partners, when they're able to look at artwork that the others have made in that circuit, we understand each other in a more

human way. So I think it's important that we look at the work of people with a diagnosis to acknowledge the fact that these people are still important. They're still capable and they're still human beings that, like every other human being, has the right to be respected and human dignity and all those things. That they are still valuable members of society.

So that's one thing and I also think that the others, the care partners at home, the family members at home and the professionals, the nurses and the doctors and everything, I really believe it's important that those two aspects of this constellation, they should be making art too because I think reflecting on our relationships and digesting what it means to care for someone else and care for ourselves is very important. I think that it's unfortunately common for care partners to get swallowed up by the intensity of the care and the monotony of the care, and it's hard. I think making artwork allows the people in this group to rejuvenate themselves and express themselves in a positive way that can be discussed and there can be a discourse about their experiences in a positive way.

I think for me, too often, I've been in a lot of support groups and things like that and there's a lot of negative ways we can handle our experiences and I can't live there. I can't live in a negative space and see all the bad things and that kind of blocks out the value of our relationships, which is the most important part of, you know, any situation, including having a diagnosis. So I think by creating artwork, whatever it is, whether it's dancing in the kitchen or writing a poem, any of the arts, it's a way of getting in touch with a different part of yourself that's a reflection and digestion of your experience, I think. It's a positive thing. And it helps people understand their humanity and what it means to be a person.

Colin Ward, former civil servant

The final contribution is from Colin Ward. Colin decided to do a number of things once he received his diagnosis of Alzheimer's disease and posterior cortical atrophy (PCA), including participation in numerous research studies (National Institute for Health Research, 2017). One of them was to agree to meet me and to speak to university students about his experiences of life lived with dementia. Irene, Colin's wife, was totally supportive and also accompanied Colin on at least one occasion. In the passage below, Colin explains why he decided to speak to students and what he got out of it:

> *Colin:* I think it's a follow-up, follow, follow-on from how I've always been at work. I was always somebody at the forefront of everything, anything new as well, and this disease that I'm struck with, it's relatively new and I don't think enough people are aware of, of what it's like to suffer dementia in all its forms, and especially if you've got two sorts like I have – one extremely rare – and people can't believe when I start speaking that I've got dementia, for a kick off, which is a big fillip for me. It means that I look and sound normal, which is how I want to be. But, of course, I can't be because I can't, I can't think straight, I can't act properly all the time, I need help with different things where, which are a constant problem for me, in my wellbeing, because I have to rely on this girl here, my wife, for all sorts of things that came normally to me that are no longer there.

> *DR:* And you talk about this being in keeping with how you've always been, with leading?

> *Colin:* Yes.

> *DR:* What do you mean by that then? Is it about the teaching

and agreeing to be involved in teaching? Is that about being prepared to be the one to take responsibility?

Colin: Yes. That's why I got on so well or so quickly anyway at the [Civil Service]. Because I was always willing to be there if somebody wanted me, it might be from another section that'd walk into our group and ask questions and they always knew they could come to me and I'll help them if I could, and usually I could. And, I've used that all the way through my life, really, whether it's leading a darts team for instance, I was always at the front of that! I've only just thought about that one [laughs]. Playing rugby, I was always the one to go to, kick the goals, that sort of thing.

DR: How do you feel when you've done the teaching though? Does it give you...

Colin: A big, big fillip!

DR: Tell me more about that. I think people would be interested to know more about that.

Colin: Well, it's like, I suppose, I'm not religious but it must be like somebody who goes into church to get absolved from something or other – what's the word I'm looking for?

DR: I think that's the right word.

Colin: And that, this is the sort of kick I get from it, erm, I feel as if I've done some good, especially if I can tell somebody else what it's like to have this incapacity because it's such a terrible affliction.

DR: And you've said this to me in person when we've finished teaching as well, you've been quite elated I think.

Colin: I have, it's, it's like casting off, casting off some of the stigma of Alzheimer's because it's still, to this day, people think you're doolally, because you've got Alzheimer's. And, I take, every time I talk to a stranger – in other words – stranger to me, I nearly always hit them big saying 'Well, I've got Alzheimer's' and then they look at you and I've been talking to them for maybe a few minutes about whatever it is we're there for and they look aghast sometimes, and then I say, 'Well not only that but I've got two sorts, one of them's called PCA'. 'Oh, what's that?' 'Posterior cortical atrophy.' When I come out with that, right enough, they go 'Ohh!...' In a way for me what I've developed, because you've given me the opportunity to talk to students especially, what I've developed is a way of dealing with dementia and it's a big relief. Every time I speak to somebody that I've never met before, and I do a lot [laughs], I think they've learnt something new but I've also got a big kick out of it by being able to show them that you might have this incapacity but you're not out of this world. You're still here and you're still operating.

What I have learned most of all from the time I have spent speaking with people who have dementia is that my expectations are always wrong. The people I have had the honour of meeting and listening to are thoughtful, resilient, knowledgeable, experienced, insightful and surprising. They have been generous in teaching me about their lives and have enriched my life in so many ways through friendship, good humour and support. I have also had to unlearn what I thought I knew about dementia and where expertise is to be found. I'm pleased to be able to namecheck some of my teachers. Finally, Pat Sikes recently suggested to me that an indication of progress in public understanding of dementia is that today some persons with dementia are almost like 'popstars', they are so well known (Sikes, 2020). Perhaps if greater credit was given to more persons with dementia for what they can do, it wouldn't be seen as so exceptional for those with the most credible understanding of dementia to be educating us.

Summary

In this chapter, the focus has been on learning from persons with dementia. The educational perspective associated with this view of relationship-centred dementia care is writ large in the identification of the significant role persons with dementia have and have had in changing society's views of dementia, albeit largely without credit. A call is made to address this appropriation of expertise. Some key moments are noted in changing ideas about dementia and an argument is made that the seat of expertise in dementia has shifted from its traditional home in universities to organisations by and for persons with dementia. In keeping with Post's (2001) ideas about an epistemology of humility in dementia, care and support practitioners are asked to identify when and what they have learned from persons with dementia, to give credit where this is due. Personal examples of learning from persons with dementia are described, identifying insights about the significance of who sets the agenda for learning and what is learned, ideas about the qualities persons with dementia want from care and support practitioners, the power of art and creativity for everyone in the dementia 'constellation' to understand their shared humanity and, finally, the new teaching careers that can open up for persons with dementia when they are given opportunities to educate others.

In the following chapter, attention turns to what practitioners can learn from family members and supporters.

CHAPTER 3

Learning from Family Members and Supporters

Introduction

In the relationship-centred approach that I am outlining, the second main 'group' that care practitioners must learn from consists of family members and supporters. They, along with persons with dementia and dementia care practitioners themselves, are key participants in episodes of dementia care and support. The same critical approach described in the previous chapter is also required in thinking about family members and supporters, and the expertise they possess. For example, have you noticed that I have avoided using the word 'carers' to describe family members and others who provide care and support to persons with dementia? Can you think why I have done this?

The layout and content of this chapter is influenced by some advice I received when I was planning a new dementia education course (Reid and Witherspoon, 2008). I organised a focus group of persons with dementia and their family members to seek their opinions about what I should include in this course and why. The overwhelming message they communicated was that dementia care practitioners on the proposed course should be given opportunities to 'walk in our footsteps' in order to understand more clearly what impact dementia has on the lives of those affected directly. In this chapter, 'walking in their footsteps' is deployed in two ways to encourage greater understanding of these experiences.

First, you are invited to read a piece of writing by a woman who provided care and support to her dad. Written specifically for this book, this account offers a variety of potential insights into the complexity of life and relationships, over time, within a family when someone has dementia and for which the label 'carer' does scant justice. Jane Watson, the author, intended that this writing would encourage a deeper appreciation among dementia care practitioners of 'caring'. It is her invitation to you to walk in her footsteps. Some possible learning outcomes from this account are suggested.

The second part of this chapter focuses on practical ways of seeking to learn from family members and supporters in your daily work and about how to offer appropriate support. Here, more is said about the range of people who find themselves with caring or support responsibilities. However, the emphasis is on developing practical ideas for learning which involve recognising, acknowledging and accessing the unique expertise possessed by family members and supporters about persons with dementia. Using the idea of 'walking in our footsteps' helps identify practical opportunities to do just that. The dementia care practitioner's role also involves a responsibility to listen to family members or supporters, and interaction with them gives you opportunities to understand their perspectives. What is learned from them can give you a good idea of their needs. This can prompt action to offer support, if providing support is a part of your role, and, regardless of your role, it will give insights to guide you when signposting family members and supporters to helpful sources of information and specialist support. A summary of possible learning from this discussion concludes the chapter.

MY DAD, JAMES, BY JANE WATSON

My dad was James Fred Earnest Hughes. My mum is Betty Francis Misen Hughes. Both my parents agreed that when they had children they would only give them one Christian name because when it comes to signing anything it becomes tedious and time consuming. I think that was really considerate of them! D is my husband, although at the time my dad developed dementia, we had only been married for eight years – relatively new to marriage.

This is a personal reflection and I appreciate that not everyone will have the same feelings or experiences: the despair, the frustrations, the very fine line between love and hate, feeling a failure because I was not able to cope, the loss of the strong person I knew as my dad – and the anticipatory grief, grieving the dad I lost from the onset of his dementia. However, living through this experience has given me insight, enabling me to truly understand how families feel when they give their loved one over to a care home as they can no longer manage through sheer frustration and exhaustion. When you are caring for someone with dementia, the future never seems to get better.

I want to talk about the role that I played when I had my dad with dementia living with us, and my mum, and what led up to that and my current work within a care home, and how I can use the feelings and experiences to help others. No one says 'Oh, Mum is going into a care home' and says it as a very positive thing, do they? What we hear is always the negative: 'She *had* to go into a care home' or 'We *had* to put him in a care home.' So, people think that's the end of their life when – and I hope to demonstrate – it can be a new beginning. It's about making a difference.

My dad was born – and I had to get this from my mother because I keep forgetting it – on 24 June 1916. He came from a family of six and he was the third child. He married my mum in 1941. His dementia started when he was 67.

I want to explain a bit about me, about my knowledge and

skills – not to sit here and say 'Look what I've done!' but rather, 'Look what I've done and I still couldn't cope!' I've been in nursing now for 38 years – quite a long time. I started work at a Yorkshire hospital but before that I was a nursing student at a Lincolnshire hospital for two years from the age of 16.

I dabbled in some work in care homes, trying to see where I'd fit, and my experience left me thinking 'Oh, never look after older people!' I didn't find it exciting, and working in care was very different then. I know you'll laugh but [for treatment of pressure sores] we would apply egg white and oxygen to bottoms – there weren't any pads – and then we'd wrap them in drawer sheets. There were no rubber gloves, and the care was pretty poor. Care was a hard word to use really. It was never seen as a positive thing, so I didn't want to go into caring for older people. Instead, I trained as an occupational health nurse and spent eight years in heavy industry, then I worked for the district nurse service in Sheffield, at Dore and Totley, which also encompassed Manor and Wybourn. It was from the sublime to the ridiculous really, the very well off to the not so well off.

During that time, I felt that I needed to develop my skills because I felt very exposed, working in somebody's house, with no team to rely on. I felt ill-equipped to deal with bereavement, death and dying when I had to do the support visits. So I did a diploma in palliative care and I then went on to do a BA honours degree. I hold the title of specialist practitioner. I studied at Master's level just to prove to myself that I could do it, but I didn't finish it and I'm too old to finish it now!

Even with all that knowledge I still struggled when my dad developed dementia. I moved to Sheffield when I was 18 but my mum lives in Lincolnshire in a tiny village, just one road in and one road out. Services there remain very poor, as it's still very much a postcode lottery. I think in all the years she's been there she's only had two GP visits at home. They have to get to the surgery by hook or by crook. She's 90 now.

So, I was living my life in Sheffield, divorced from my first husband and making a new relationship with my second husband, a totally different man altogether. D worked for 42 years for one company as a foreman. He's now retired, and is very much a manual man. Gentle, soft aren't words I'd use to describe him. We purchased a house in Sheffield but then my dad started to change, though we didn't quite know what was wrong at first.

He was a very, very strict father and liked to be totally in control of everything, including us. Firm but fair, he nurtured his family. He worked hard all his life – 25 years for British Steel, followed by 25 years for the Post Office as a postman, getting up most mornings at 3.30am. He had high standards and a good work ethic. I suppose Dad instilled those standards in his family. He was always dressed very smartly in a collar and tie, with a small well-trimmed moustache, highly polished shoes, never a hair out of place, and impeccable manners – a perfect gentleman.

He moved our family out to a small village so he could control us – there was nobody else there. We went to private Catholic school. From the age of four, we would be out at 6am on the bus to school and then not get back until after 6pm, so our day was quite nicely sorted for us really! I moved away to start my nursing career. When my dad started to become cantankerous we just thought he was getting more difficult as he got older, and it was quite hard for my mum living with him. Then certain things started to happen which sent a ripple effect through the family.

He took the dog for a walk one day and came back to the house with no dog. He'd actually left him by the graveyard where he used to stop and have his pipe of tobacco. My mum said, 'Well, where's the dog?' 'Oh, bloody hell, I don't know!' So he went out to find him. On another occasion, he decided to get up and cook his breakfast; he liked a cooked breakfast but we had polystyrene tiles and he set the house on fire! Then my mother really started to get worried. She asked for a GP visit, and as they were about to drive back he turned to my mother and said, 'So what do I do now?' And my mother doesn't drive. So, things had to be looked at really.

He was one of those men who would say, 'What happens within our house stops within our house.' Nothing was shared elsewhere. Very firm. So my mum had to find a roundabout way of getting the GP to come out and for my dad to be there for the assessment. He was a new doctor, a young doctor. He came out but he couldn't actually put his finger on what was wrong; he thought my dad had Parkinson's disease. That was his broad diagnosis at the time but suggested he would refer him to the hospital. So he left him the drugs to take. On the visit, my dad told the doctor that my mum was regularly pushing him downstairs, which was totally untrue, and she had to defend herself to the doctor, so she said, 'No, that isn't happening.'

Gradually, things became worse. I used to ring every night to find out how they were and in some ways my mother was protecting me because I was setting up a new life here and she was aware of that, but she was beginning not to cope. Then she developed shingles because she was so low in caring for my dad. It was becoming very stressful. If they had visitors to the house, as soon as they sat down, he would thank them very much for coming, get up and open the door for them to leave, which my mum found very embarrassing because at this point she didn't know why he was behaving as he was. People stopped wanting to visit because they felt embarrassed, not only for my dad but also my mum. Gradually, there were fewer and fewer visitors to the house, leaving my mum very isolated.

So things began to get considerably worse, and when my mum developed the shingles I actually brought them over to Sheffield to live with me, short term, so I could monitor what was going on with my dad. They came for a short spell, but in order to access the services he needed he had to go back to Lincolnshire. So they were swinging backwards and forwards. There was a marked deterioration in my dad. Eventually, he was assessed at Scunthorpe Hospital and discharged back home with: 'He has dementia. Look after him.' That was it. My mum felt very much on her own, isolated in her village, with a man who was becoming more aggressive – though he had never been an aggressive or violent man.

It was very hard. My mum is the best person to recount this really, as only she can say how isolated she felt, how people didn't visit her because of my dad's reaction and how he was getting more and more aggressive towards her. The man I knew as my father, who was very stern but never hit us – he only had to look, that was enough – was turning into somebody I didn't know or recognise. And my mum didn't either. There was no social worker support, no day centre support, we just had to get on and look after him. So I moved them back in again with me. That's when the reality of dad's diagnosis of dementia started to impact on the family and on the roles people played within the family unit.

In his eyes, I was his sister. I wasn't his daughter. I looked very much like his sister H. My mum is very short, but my dad was very tall and I take after him. My mum's eyes are blue, mine are brown. Dad didn't know what had happened that day, that morning, that afternoon – but was quite au fait with 50 years ago. If you travelled back 50 years you could hold a conversation about the past. He had no future and no here and now, and that was very hard. He began to get more violent, more aggressive, and he needed 24-hour care. I knew that my dad wouldn't have wanted me to put him in the bath – he was a very private man – so I used to ask my husband to do it for me. Well, D is a bit rough and ready. He's a wonderful husband and I've been with him for 33 years and I wouldn't swap him for the world, but he doesn't know how to bath anybody. I didn't take that into consideration because that was my dad, and I was going to look after him, whatever it took. I suppose, on reflection, I never took D into account. My mum had always been a good mum, she had never left me, so I was going to be a good daughter. I had a brother who only lived two miles down the road but he was having his family and he really didn't get involved. His new wife didn't want her baby near anyone with dementia, because they were unpredictable. In some ways, I could understand this, but in other ways I still find it quite difficult. So, when my dad needed a bath, I used to have to approach D and say, 'Oh, my dad really needs to get in the bath tonight, D. How are you fixed?' And he did it, begrudgingly, but he did it.

I suppose I was expecting too much of my husband – he's very caring, he'll do anything for you, but you have to tell him what to do. If you were lying in bed unwell and you asked him to fetch you a bowl of water for a wash, then he'd do it. But he wouldn't think of saying, 'Shall I get you a bowl of water so you can have a wash?' He's that kind of man. So looking back I suppose I didn't factor in his feelings. He was married to me so he was part of me, and he had to do what I asked him to do. My dad had enough awareness that when the white van turned up, meaning my husband was home, he had to behave in a very different manner, because D wouldn't tolerate it. He seemed to know not to go too far when D was in the room. He didn't know his name but he knew that D was probably my husband or he knew he had to behave in a certain way. It was strange to watch – you wouldn't believe it unless you actually saw it.

Luckily, Dad was continent, so getting him ready for bed was basically putting the pyjamas out and making sure he didn't tumble over. We'd get him into bed at 9pm and breathe a sigh of relief and think 'Phew! It's our time now...', a bit like you do when you have small kids. But then two minutes later the door would open, and it would be: 'What are you doing, burning this electricity?'

And he would start turning the television off, and turning the lights off. D had been at work all day and became less and less tolerant of this behaviour.

And, bless him, D had no understanding and he thought that my dad was doing it deliberately: 'He knows what he's doing! He wouldn't be able to do *that* if he can do that!' It got to a point where my mum sensed that it was causing quite a lot of friction in the house. At 4am Dad would get up, wash and dress because he was a postman. He was in his routine. There was one toilet in the house and he occupied it. D would be trying to get to work, with seven men to pick up, whose wages he was responsible for, because if he didn't pick them up, they didn't get paid. So the pressure was building and building in the pot, and something had to give.

When we got him to our house, I took what must have been between six and seven thousand pounds from his pocket, which he wouldn't let anybody have. It was in his wallet, because he always controlled everything. He paid the bills. My mother got housekeeping money and that was it. No good on Tuesday saying, 'I've run out of money.' She had to manage. He paid everything; he looked after everything. So, not only was I having to deal with my dad, who was going downhill, but my mum also, who was mentally and physically exhausted. I tried to get her to be independent, and start looking at how to manage opening a bank account. So there were these two elements running at the same time, and I was trying to keep the cart on the wheels with D, who thought Dad was doing it all deliberately, when he really wasn't! I hadn't got enough knowledge at that point to manage that situation but I was determined to look after my dad no matter what.

One day he went to the local shop, got a bottle of syrup of figs, drunk it and locked himself in the toilet for two days. Of course, none of us could get in. The frustration behind that was unbelievable! I'd given the instruction to the shop to 'let him have what he wants and I'll come and settle up with you'; 'if he comes for his paper, if he comes for his cigarettes or his pipe tobacco – let him have it'. And they did that exactly – they were lovely. It's funny now to laugh at that story, and if my dad hadn't had his dementia – he had a wonderful sense of humour – he would have found that story quite funny too.

The day came when we had to look at 24-hour care because, gradually, all of us were sinking. D felt very neglected and pushed out because I put this other man, my father, in front of him. My mum was trying to keep the cart on the wheels because she knew my dad was being a nuisance, as she called him, and upsetting things in the house, so we had to look at how we were going to manage.

Eventually, he went into a care home in Lincolnshire. It was a long process. I think when the care home saw me coming it was a bit like 'Oh my God! Hide! Scatter!' because I was not happy with what I saw. I've now got a wiser head on my shoulders, but at that time, that was my dad and I wanted the best for him. The day he moved into the care home he stood and cried, telling me he would behave if I would take him home. That was the first time in my life that I had seen my dad cry. I will never forget that day and it still haunts me.

I would go into the care home and find he was unshaven. 'You have not bothered to put a tie on him! That's *my* dad, that's how I know my dad. And I'm walking in here and there's all you sat round having coffee and you've left him, like *that*!' So, I'd get hold of him and we'd go to the bedroom and out would come the razor and I'd shave him and present him the way I knew he would want to be presented. But thinking about it, was it for him or was it for me? I don't know, and to this day I still don't know – probably a bit of both. I wanted some semblance of how he had been.

But by the time our family needed the care home, we were all exhausted, we felt like failures. I felt a failure. And then I walked through the door and saw him looking dishevelled, and under my care he had never looked like that. It's very hard but I didn't consider that, maybe, my dad would do more for me than he would for people and strangers he didn't know. So I didn't take on board that it might have been difficult for those care staff to actually approach him, because I was a lot younger then and I didn't know as much as I do now.

So I went in and I was really very upset and I think I showed how upset I was. As I say, scattering staff, with them thinking, 'There'll be something not right, I imagine!' I say the same things myself at work now.

He was only in there a very short time and he developed a chest infection. He was the fittest out of his family – they all died from a stroke – and he would cycle on average 50 miles a day, no problems whatsoever. He liked a smoke and he liked his pipe of tobacco and he was as thin as a rake. I'd never known him have an antibiotic in his life, because he had had nearly a total gastrectomy in the past, so antibiotics weren't on his radar really. Eventually he died with the chest infection and I never pursued it; I never pushed for another doctor's visit or some different medicine. It's hard looking back. I know it affected me quite a lot. When I started to learn about palliative and terminal care later, I understood that I was going through anticipatory grief, going through a grieving process, before my dad had died. I organised my dad's funeral. I remember being at the funeral and taking the lead because that's how I'd been brought up. At the private Catholic school that I went to, the school and the church were together, so we had to go to all the funerals. I've been to so many funerals of people I didn't know – maybe three a week – and I knew how to behave because that was the way the school was set up. I don't know what effect that has had on me, but I don't go to funerals now. (I tell them it's written into my job contract. 'I can't go, due to favouritism.' I don't know quite where that's written but there we are. I don't go to funerals.)

I didn't shed a tear. I came out and I thought, 'God, you're hard! You're so hard!' I could see these people looking at me in the village. It was a wonderful funeral and the streets were lined and the pallbearers walked in front. It couldn't have been any better put together. But I had to be the strong one who kept everyone else together. I was probably the little professor from the age of about five, and I couldn't let my dad down.

Maybe five years later, I'd moved home, I was ironing away, and I turned around and I saw a bunch of daffodils, and I was heartbroken, because my dad was a keen gardener. He loved his garden. I was absolutely heartbroken. [At home] the other night I walked in and they were doing the Daffodil Appeal [on TV] and I was at it again! Twenty-five years on! I still have that emotion and I still feel that I let him down. There is a part of me that says 'You didn't!', but even though I'd got my mum to consider and a husband to consider, I was a nurse, and I cared for people with dementia, but I couldn't care for my own dad. It was hard to move on from that.

I hope that, if anything, it now makes me better understand how relatives feel when they come into the care home. I hope that there is a difference I can make because I can't change what happened but I can change what happens in the future. That's what I'm now trying to do. Yes, it was very hard, but anticipatory grief is – you start grieving for the person you've lost, it's a *bereavement* from losing the person that you knew. People are grieving when they're putting somebody in a care home, or their loved one comes into hospital. They've lost the person that was their mum, their dad or whoever. That's the point when you actually start to grieve. But again, no one told me about anticipatory grief, and there were times when I hated my father because I was as trapped as he was trapped.

I couldn't leave the house even to go shopping because my mum was frightened to death to be left with him – and D would say, 'Have you not been to the shops?' 'How can I?!' So, you can imagine, it was these little things in life that affected us and, I'm not ashamed to say it, but there was a very fine line between love and hate. My dad never told me he loved me. Ever. But I know he loved me. He didn't have to tell me, that was the kind of relationship we had. He was very loyal to me and I was very loyal to him. He always used to say things that I would never achieve – to get the best out of me and, maybe, I am the person today because he made me a stronger person.

I decided to write this because it might make somebody change just *one thing* that they do in their approach or their realisation when a relative confronts them and is really angry, that people have been through a heck of a lot before they ever get near the care home or hospital.

If there is just one change, one comment, or someone has reassessed the way they work or gained a better understanding, then I've made a difference – and my dad has made a difference.

He hasn't got a voice now, only through me. The first few times I talked about this I found it extremely difficult but extremely cleansing as well. It still sits there, and I can get very emotional about it, because I feel I failed him. I know I haven't but I feel I have. That's why I decided to share my experience. I feel very privileged to be asked to contribute to this book. My aim is to raise awareness by sharing with others my personal difficulties in managing my dad and the impact his diagnosis of dementia had on my family, warts and all, and how the experience has changed my approach when dealing with residents and their families in my current role as a care home manager.

Next steps

There is a lot to think about after reading this. There is, no doubt, much that can be taken from Jane's account to gain a richer understanding of the experiences of family members and supporters. In the second part of this chapter, I identify what I consider to be some of the main learning points. The aim, however, is not to encourage generalisations. This is Jane's account. Rather, the aim is to reveal the complexity of providing care and support to someone with dementia when that person is someone you love, a father, mother, brother, sister, and, as Jane herself highlights, the ripples this causes across the family and social dynamics.

The way I would like to develop this appreciation and identify ways it can lead to positive, practical action is to return to the idea that dementia care and support practitioners can orientate themselves towards learning from the expertise of family members and supporters. *What* can be learned is indicated in Jane's account, but let's focus on *why* you are seeking to learn it. One reason is that you want to learn more about the person with dementia so that you are able to offer that person care and support that is as good as it can be. Family members and supporters can possess detailed biographical knowledge about the person, as well as their likes and dislikes. If the person is unable to convey this information themselves, because of impairments associated with dementia, or for any other reason, then this knowledge may only be available from family members and supporters.

A second reason is that you want to know more about the family member or supporter and their experiences of dementia. In order to be able to offer or direct meaningful support to these people you must seek to discover their needs. In both cases, there is then a challenge to think about *how* to learn from family members and supporters and then to consider what *action* to take with the knowledge that is gained. It is to these questions that attention now turns.

Family members and supporters: their expertise and their support

There are estimated to be around 700,000 family members and supporters caring for persons with dementia in the UK (Alzheimer's Research UK, 2018). There are rich and diverse resources available relating to the experiences of family members and supporters who provide care and support to persons with dementia. I do not attempt to summarise it here but do suggest strongly that you explore the huge range of research studies (e.g. Brodaty and Donkin, 2009; Royal Surgical Aid Society, 2016; Sikes and Hall, 2018; Greenwood and Smith, 2019), videos (e.g. Healthtalk.org, 2018), information sources (e.g. Social Care Institute for Excellence, 2015b; Age UK, 2020a), free online courses (e.g. Social Care Institute for Excellence, 2019) and online communities aimed at all 'carers' (e.g. Carers UK, 2020a) or those specifically for those supporting persons with dementia (e.g. 'Dementia Talking Point' – see Alzheimer's Society, 2020c; see also YoungDementia UK, 2019).

For current purposes, it is important to note that there has been an interest in these experiences and perspectives for many years, as there has been in improving carers' rights, generally. Though progress has been slow, carers' rights have extended into employment and other areas, and knowing about these rights can help you empower family members and supporters of persons with dementia. A useful starting point for understanding carers' rights is provided by Caring for the Carers (2020).

Another way that 'walking in our footsteps' helps practitioners think more about learning from family members and supporters is to visualise the opportunities you typically have to speak with them when they contact, enter, spend time in and then leave the dementia care or support environment. You literally map those key points at which you or members of your team usually encounter family carers and supporters in your setting. You could choose to take an 'audit' approach and simply compile a list of typical interactions. This might be best done as a team task so that interactions you are unaware of, because it's not part of your role, are picked up, too.

The contents of the list will, of course, vary from setting to setting. Some dementia care practitioners will have multiple typical interactions, others may have relatively few. For example, at a community-based activity or service, such as a dementia cafe or choir, family members and supporters might well be attending themselves and are therefore available for the duration of the session. In care homes, family members and supporters may have a regular and predictable pattern of attendance and may also be in touch intermittently over the telephone or by email. In acute clinical care settings, there may be very few opportunities for interaction and the majority of contact is in the form of brief, snatched, conversations in corridors or over the telephone. So, your own list will, to a large degree, reflect the purpose of your service or activity.

This first step in identifying typical learning opportunities has the benefit of making visible an important activity which might go on informally, is under-recognised and, consequently, might be undervalued. By doing this it is then possible to think about what happens to the information that is learned during these interactions. Is it written down? Is it shared? Is it simply remembered by individuals and used by them as 'working knowledge'? Of course, many dementia care and support services use the 'This is me' leaflet (Alzheimer's Society, 2020d), a standardised form for obtaining information about the person with dementia to aid, among other things, effective communication. Other approaches, such as a Healthcare Passport (Leavey, Corry, Curren *et al.*, 2017) and, significantly, the Carer Passport Scheme (Carers UK, 2020b), offer great potential for ensuring carers' needs are identified and met in health care settings.

The intention behind the 'This is me' form is to enable

practitioners to obtain key information about the person which can then be shared easily to help ensure that the person with dementia's preferences, needs and key biographical information – including identification of 'the carers/people who know me best' – are known by all. How this form is completed varies, but one way is for it to be completed with the dementia care practitioner present, who may learn some additional information in the course of conversation. Many practitioners have told me that they find the 'This is me' form very helpful, in particular, when the person with dementia is unable to communicate verbally as a result of cognitive impairment or illness. For the family member or supporter, it must also be a valuable resource, offering the potential means by which care practitioners know something of the person with whom they are entrusted.

If you do use the 'This is me' form, a critical question to ask, as part of a discussion about learning from family members and supporters, is whether or not you and your team are using the information it contains about *them*, as well as using the information about the person with dementia. Is the form being completed for every person with dementia? Is the completed form made accessible to all staff colleagues to read and use? Is what is learned about the family member or supporter shared and, on the basis of this information, are they offered any form of support by you or your team? Having a form to complete provides a focal point for information collection. While the 'This is me' document does provide some space to prompt questions and record information about family and supporters, it is really orientated towards the person with dementia. In my view, the Carer Passport (Carers UK, 2020b) offers a much more comprehensive approach to ensuring that carers' needs are being assessed.

Completion of forms does not represent the only times when dementia care practitioners have opportunities to learn from family members and supporters. It might be that, alongside the opportunities you have already identified, or among them, there are scheduled relatives' or carers' groups. Many residential and nursing homes attempt to facilitate these groups and, while they can be poorly attended, such groups offer family members the chance to share their views and expertise. While some things may be more appropriate or practicable when shared one-to-one, groups provide spaces where people may feel empowered, having the moral support of others available, to raise issues or disclose information which dementia care practitioners benefit from knowing.

Of course, family members and supporters are not only able to offer insights about the person they care for and a commentary on how they are managing or coping – both of which can be turned into action. Family members and supporters are in ongoing relationships with their loved ones – and vice versa (Graham and Bassett, 2006). They may provide intelligence to you, but the act of sharing is not a signal that they have stopped being in relationships with the person with dementia. For the past few years, John's Campaign (2020; Age UK, 2020b) has sought to make it easier for family members and supporters to remain with their loved one while they are accessing acute health care settings, and a growing number of NHS trusts have signed up to the campaign's demands. Has your NHS trust?

The basis of John's Campaign is dissatisfaction among family members and supporters about the restrictions imposed on their ability to be with their loved ones by the excesses of what might be called the 'visiting hours' culture. Notwithstanding global pandemics and specific and justifiable restrictions on visiting associated with infection control and clinical priorities, the existence of narrow visiting hours places undue restrictions on family and supporters, impacting their ability to maintain their relationships. In many cases, restricted visiting hours are simply a hangover from a different era, where such regimentation was in place mainly to serve a task-oriented culture of care. John's Campaign (2020) argues that by 'allowing' family members and supporters to have greater fluidity of access to acute care settings, they can provide company, social interaction, maintenance of family life and a host of other benefits to the person with dementia and to the staff team. For example, where staff–patient ratios in acute settings can be overwhelming, family carers and supporters can make a positive difference. There is a free-to-download guide called *Implementing John's Campaign* available for practitioners (John's Campaign, 2020).

Meeting the needs of family members and supporters requires some effort to identify what these needs are and, importantly, a clear idea about what support might be practicable to offer. There are clearly a number of opportunities for you to discover who family members and supporters are and to learn what they know about the person with dementia. It should go without saying that the person with dementia is the expert in their own experience. Yet, equally, the family member or supporter has their own experience of dementia, too. The special role of the dementia care practitioner is to be able to recognise and work with the fact that the person with dementia and their family member or supporter may have different experiences of life lived with dementia. It is not necessary to choose one over the other; both are to be valued.

In communication with both, at different times, these differences might be quite glaring. The point, I argue, is not to focus on weighing up and deciding whose description of the person with dementia is most accurate, precise and credible. This way of thinking sets up an unnecessary competition and can seriously undermine the person with dementia. Understanding the experiences of the person with dementia requires learning from both the person and the family member or supporter. How you do this will depend largely on you and your 'experience of dementia', which is the focus of the next chapter. Both the person with dementia and the family member or supporter have needs which it is your role to discern.

Focusing now not on learning about the person with dementia but on the needs of family members and supporters, it should be clear that there are various opportunities to do this. Simply asking 'How are you?' when the opportunity arises can provide family members and supporters with the chance to share with you very useful information. It has already been noted that some settings simply do not offer chances to spend time doing this, either because of clinical priorities, restricted access hours or because staff–patient ratios do not allow it. Initiatives such as 'This is me', the Carer Passport or carers' and relatives' groups can provide structured opportunities to discover how well or not family members and supporters are coping.

There are both formal and informal ways of learning about the experiences of family members and supporters, and a first challenge, therefore, is to identify what these are. The reason for giving this emphasis, for prioritising it, should be obvious from reflecting on Jane's account. The informal and formal chances to talk to staff are vital for family members and supporters to share what they know, to be reassured that you know their loved one and, quite reasonably, to maintain an active relationship with that person. It is notable that during the Covid-19 pandemic, many dementia care and support practitioners have excelled in doing just that, often at great personal risk and sacrifice (Guardian, 2020b).

There is more to learn by putting yourself in the place of family members and supporters because through this learning it is possible to prepare yourself by anticipating the possible emotive and anxious behaviour which might emerge during these interactions, be they fleeting and informal, or structured, formal discussions. Family members and supporters have a right and expectation to maintain a relationship with their loved one. Wouldn't you? This holds true even when they are no longer living in the same place because, for example, the impairments associated with a person's dementia become too severe for normal family and social life to continue.

Drawing on Jane's account, here are some further suggestions to be made about needs and you are invited to add to them from your own reading. First, family members and supporters may not understand dementia and how it affects individuals. Second, the impact of dementia often includes social isolation for those without dementia (Greenwood, Mezey and Smith, 2018). Third, knowing who to contact and how to access support can be problematic, particularly for black and minority ethnic carers of persons with dementia (Johl, Patterson and Pearson, 2016). Fourth, dementia affects a number of people across families, including children (Sikes and Hall, 2018), and within social networks. Finally, the emotional and psychological impact of dementia can be complex and, in relation to grief, may endure for years after a person with dementia has died (Chan, Livingston, Jones *et al.*, 2013).

This is by no means an exhaustive list but comes simply from an attempt to think about how family members and supporters experience dementia. Each person will be different. I do not suggest that you and your colleagues must become experts in identifying and supporting the needs of family members and supporters. That would be inappropriate, unrealistic and unnecessary. Such specialised support is available elsewhere. Instead, there is, I argue, a basic requirement to ensure that all family members and supporters are valued, listened to and learned from, encouraged to maintain relationships with their loved ones, with unjustifiable barriers removed so that these people can be with their loved ones when they want. I believe there is also a requirement to ensure that you are able to signpost family members and supporters to credible local and national organisations and sources of advice and information which might assist them in having their own unique needs met.

A simple starting point for a practical way of meeting the needs of family members and supporters is to ask: what information and advice is currently possessed that we could give them? Providing information and advice is not a substitute for interacting with family members and supporters – it is an addition to this. If your staff team does not have information and advice available, why is this? What would you include within this resource? Is there already a geographically specific carer information booklet available? Could you ask family members and supporters for their recommendations? Are there organisations in your town or city that deal specifically with carers' needs, such as a carers' centre? Are there sources of support, such as carers' peer support groups, organised by the Alzheimer's Society or Age UK, which have a specific dementia remit? Who is going to put this information together into something that can be given to family members and supporters? When is it going to be reviewed and updated? The *Sheffield Dementia Information Pack* is one such resource (Reid, Warnes and Low, 2014; Reid, 2019).

There are many questions. However, an initial contact information sheet containing signposts to sources of information, advice and support for family members and supporters could be compiled fairly quickly. This could become the basis for developing something more comprehensive, over time. In this process, opportunities are created for you to develop partnerships with relevant local organisations. My own experience of helping to establish and then coordinate the *Sheffield Dementia Information Pack* is that there are more organisations than you realise for people to contact. There is also a thirst for this kind of signposting information. An accurate list, with contact details and websites, of key statutory and voluntary sector organisations with responsibilities for family members and supporters of persons with dementia (usually referred to as 'carers') is a modest and realistic project for a busy dementia care and support service. By being more attentive to the needs of these essential partners in care and support, you can connect people with other experts best placed to assess and meet their diverse needs.

Summary

This chapter has been an invitation to walk in the footsteps of family members and supporters. It is an invitation to value and learn from their expertise. Their expertise can help you realise or remember that family members and supporters remain in their relationships with the person with dementia – unique relationships like you and I have with our loved ones. This understanding can help you to anticipate how family members and supporters might feel when they meet you and appreciate better why they retain a keen concern with the person's welfare and want to or must remain involved, if given the chance.

You have been asked to audit the typical opportunities family members and supporters have to share their knowledge and perspectives in your dementia care or support setting, and consider critically what happens to that intelligence. You have been challenged to consider what information and advice to offer to family members and supporters to ensure that they have what they require to make contact, should they wish to, with others like them or links to resources and organisations which might assess and meet their individual needs. In the next chapter, attention turns to you, the dementia care practitioner, and an examination of the vital, personal, role you play in *doing* relationship-centred dementia care. You, like persons with dementia, family members and supporters, have your own unique experience of dementia, too, and it matters.

CHAPTER 4

Dementia Care and Support Practitioners' Experiences of Dementia

Introduction

Each dementia care practitioner has their own 'experiences of dementia'. In this chapter, an attempt is made to explain what this means and how awareness of this experience can help you in the relationship-centred dementia care and support that you lead. First, some dimensions of your 'personal' experience of dementia are suggested and an argument is made for why exploring this is overdue. Second, there is a focus on the special leadership role which each practitioner has in episodes of dementia care and support. This form of leadership relates to your learning from both persons with dementia and from family members and supporters. Some of the challenges and obstacles facing dementia care and support practitioners are identified.

To develop a greater appreciation and understanding of the practitioner's 'personal' experience of dementia, I draw on ideas that originate in conversations I have shared with dementia care and support practitioners. As a result of these ideas, it is suggested that there are 'private', 'public' and 'practical' dimensions to your personal experience of dementia. Towards the end of the chapter, some possible links between your own personal experiences of dementia and the ways you approach and engage in your work are discussed. Key learning from this discussion is taken forwards and explored in more detail in Chapters 5–7.

Lead participant

You may have noticed throughout this book so far that the dementia care and support practitioner has not only been positioned as an active participant in dementia care and support but as the lead participant. The idea of 'lead participant' is simply to make it clear who has responsibility in the communications that go on in and around care and support practice. As lead participant, I argue you have a responsibility to view interactions with both persons with dementia and family members and supporters as educational, as opportunities to learn from their expertise, their experiences of life lived with dementia – whatever that aspect of life it is you are all attending to.

Each practitioner has their job to do. Some of you reading this may have infrequent contact with persons with dementia, others daily contact. Some will have jobs, roles and responsibilities which are predominantly clinical, where the focus is on treating illness in specialist medical settings. Others will have jobs in community-based settings where your role is to facilitate individual or group activities. Still others will work in group home-like environments where your role may combine medical and social responsibilities.

Wherever you work and whatever the priorities, there will be a common need for someone to communicate with the person with dementia and their family member or supporter intermittently or throughout their engagement with that service. That person is you. But should it really matter *which* practitioner a person with dementia encounters, or who a family member or supporter speaks with? Well, going back to the ideas from persons with dementia and family members who were asked for what practitioners should learn on a dementia educational course (Chapter 2), there is a strong indication that it does matter, whether or not it should. It does matter. Quality of communication matters in all things. However, it arguably matters significantly more in dementia care and support because of the uncertainty that accompanies dementia. Being able and willing to communicate effectively with persons with dementia and their family members and supporters cannot be taken for granted.

Is it possible to claim that anyone *is* an effective communicator with persons with dementia? The diversity of persons with dementia militates against such a bold presumption. This is not about absolutes or prizes. Also, everyone makes mistakes or gets it wrong on occasions and this is, of course, when learning can occur. That said, beginning to consider what qualities make for an effective communicator is no bad thing. This is a positive move because rather than reducing communication skills to pointing fingers at the person with dementia and their impairments – a reductive approach – it turns the focus more fully on you, the individual dementia care and support practitioner. There do seem to be some who have or develop skills and understanding which mean that they are able to be with persons with dementia and their family members and supporters, to listen and to learn, in the midst of the uncertainties faced by those to whom they offer care and support and, quite likely, their own uncertainties. But, for everyone, learning how to do this effectively is ongoing.

The sort of leadership that I am suggesting each dementia care and support practitioner takes is, first and foremost, in relation to their personal interactions with persons with dementia, family members and supporters. This is not the full extent of leadership which might be possible, and more is said about other, possible forms of leadership in Chapter 6. However, it is only when you take personal responsibility as lead participant in communications with persons with dementia and family members and supporters, approaching these people as experts and with a willingness to learn, that you can be satisfied yourself that at this level you have done all that you can to understand their needs.

By striving for this kind of effective communication within the care and support relationships to which you contribute, you would be doing so not in response to someone's theory of dementia care or because it is on a list of things policy states you should do. It is simply about treating persons with dementia and their family members and supporters as knowledgeable, valuable, full human beings, adopting an attitude of humility and exercising critical thought about what's most important in dementia care and support. You are recognised to be the expert in the dementia care and support that *you* offer or provide. Humility is in accepting that others are experts in their experiences and in appreciating that learning is an ongoing process, if you choose to view it as such. Critical thought, as has been noted elsewhere, is what is required to be a thoughtful and, therefore, active consumer of dementia knowledge. Importantly, this includes reflecting on your own communication approach, and being willing and able to adapt, develop and innovate.

In the ideas about relationship-centred dementia care outlined here, you are considered capable of critical thought, empathy, reflection, highly skilled communication, research skills, advocacy – but also, and underpinning all of these, a desire to provide the highest quality of care and support that is possible. However, when your own expertise and your ways of doing dementia care and support in practice are largely ignored, when you, the person who does dementia care and support, is devalued, then I believe it is not possible to have a meaningful debate about how dementia care and support can be improved.

To develop a greater appreciation and understanding of

the practitioner's personal experience of dementia I now draw on some ideas that originate with dementia care and support practitioners. There have been a number of occasions when I have explored this idea of 'personal experience of dementia' directly with practitioners in the classroom. It should be noted that it was practitioners themselves who first prompted me to think more about the potential significance of this to care and support practice, and they did this consistently in discussions we shared during the large number of dementia awareness study days and other courses I have facilitated.

From these discussions, I learned that dementia care and support practitioners had what I describe as 'private' experiences of dementia and 'practical' experiences of dementia – components of their personal experience of dementia – which seemed to have a bearing on how they approached doing dementia care and support. You will see in what follows that it is sometimes difficult to make an easy distinction between the two. In the next section, I provide an account of how both of these types of personal experience of dementia (i.e. the 'private' and the 'practical') were first described to me by practitioners in dementia awareness study days. For each, the private and the practical experiences of dementia, I share some more detailed responses from other dementia care and support practitioners who, in different education sessions I ran later, were asked directly about their personal experiences of dementia.

Private experiences of dementia

The content and structure of dementia awareness study days I ran changed a little over the years. Those who attended were usually drawn from a range of different practice settings and so did not necessarily know each other or work together on a daily basis. Over time, some content was updated and, on any given day, I might choose to vary the order in which I introduced different topics, depending on what I thought might work best for the specific group, as well as in response to various information technology contingencies.

A consistent element of the dementia awareness study day was to discuss with the group members the sorts of challenges they each faced in their particular practice settings and how they went about their roles. In these discussions, across many study days, I began to notice that a similar phrase, a sentiment, was being repeated: 'you treat people as you would want to be treated yourself'. It is a commonly heard sentiment and I think, because of this, I didn't pay much attention to it the first few times I heard it. Then, I began to wonder if practitioners do actively imagine that they are caring for or supporting *themselves* when they interact with persons with dementia.

I began to challenge practitioners a little harder on this matter, and then a couple of interesting things happened. First, some practitioners began speaking about their own lives and recounting stories of loved ones who currently or had previously had dementia. Some of these kinds of accounts are given later in this section. Second, and most arrestingly, I frequently heard practitioners muse about what they would want to happen to them should they develop dementia later in their lives. Maybe it's surprising, maybe it's not, but it was not at all uncommon for some practitioners in each session to say 'I'd take some tablets' or 'I'd end it' or words to that effect.

I would sit and listen and then say what I write now. I find it utterly amazing that practitioners who spoke both passionately and positively about wanting to ensure persons with dementia receive the best possible care and support did so while simultaneously feeling such utter dread about dementia. This resonates with Kitwood's (1997a, p.113) ideas about 'organizational defences' and feeling as if you have to hide how you feel when working with persons with dementia. Yet, when you have thought about developing dementia and it fills you with dread, then when facing a person with dementia, your interaction with that person might be affected by 'sensing' your own possible future.

What stayed with me was the sense that many practitioners must expend considerable amounts of emotional labour trying to balance the desire and commitment to offer care and support, with an instinctive horror that the prospect of developing dementia evokes within them. Given this was a sentiment which was not universally expressed, I do not want to labour this particular point. However, what seems to be suggested is that, in their work, some dementia care and support practitioners are guided or, perhaps, influenced by their private experiences, some of which are linked to imagining what living with dementia must be like and some of which relate to loved ones who have had or have dementia. That it would be healthy for practitioners to talk about such matters, and have access to appropriate support themselves, was also suggested.

Later, for another dementia education course, I had more time to explore these ideas about a personal experience of dementia with a number of cohorts of dementia care and support practitioners. I prompted their consideration by asking individuals or groups, depending on the cohort, to respond to general questions about what I now call private experiences of dementia, how they became interested in dementia care and support, and how these experiences might link to their care and support practice. Quotes from some of these practitioners' written responses are presented below for you to read and consider. It is important to remember that these should be read with an appreciation of how and when they were written, that is, on a particular day and on a particular course and knowing that I could use their responses in a publication. Therefore, I suggest the views expressed should be interpreted lightly, as indicative rather than definitive, in terms of any links they might suggest between private experience and their actual dementia care and support practice. I have no empirical evidence that their actual practice was influenced by their private experiences of dementia.

The first excerpt is from Rob, who explained how and why he came to be working as a dementia care and support practitioner. Rob identified his relationship with his grandparents as being a significant catalyst and, as he described why he enjoys working with persons with dementia, he touched on themes other practitioners refer to in their accounts:

> I first became interested in working with older people after my grandparents experienced a decline in health. This led to a change of career for me, with the aim of helping older people in their everyday lives. After working as a carer with persons with dementia, I found that I enjoyed this aspect of health care as it required challenging, interesting and compassionate skills as well as an understanding of human relationships, emotions and difficulties. I constantly find this area of work challenging and surprising as no two people are the same and I find I have to adapt myself and my responses in order to provide the care. This also brings an element of excitement to the job as I am lucky enough to have the opportunity to work with some very interesting people who have lived very rich lives, to develop relationships with them and hopefully offer some guidance and help on their journey as well as ease some distress. No two days are the same. After leaving school with no idea of what I wanted to do with my life it all became clear at 30 when I started working in dementia care. (Rob)

Alison felt that her approach to dementia care and support practice was influenced, to some degree, by her feelings of 'guilt' about her inability to do anything about her dad's illness and by an appreciation of the impact dementia had on relatives and friends:

> My personal experience of dementia has now made me look at people with dementia in a more holistic way, making me much more aware of the thoughts and feelings of, not just the patient

with dementia, but also relatives and friends. My personal feeling of 'guilt' – as a nurse, I could not make my dad better – still at times haunts me now. Continuity of care providers/professionals is paramount for individuals to receive the care and understanding that they need/deserve. Staff in homes being honest and very open to suggestions to make their environments more dementia friendly must be an added bonus. Support *must* be there not only for the person with dementia but for their family, especially their spouses. Having and making time for one-to-one care makes such a big difference for individuals. Just because a person has dementia does not mean they are not understanding what we are saying to them. (Alison)

Other practitioners were clear that personal reflection assists them in developing empathy for persons with dementia:

Your own ageing experiences help to understand how they are feeling and how you yourself would like to be treated. (Jayne, Jane, Michelle, Stacey)

There was also a similar acknowledgement from a group of practitioners that the ways they approach care and support for persons with dementia link with personally held views of how they and their families would wish to be treated:

In our personal experiences of dementia, we have found that several things have influenced us. We all agree that we should treat people how we would like us and our family to be treated if in that situation. We feel that these views have arisen from personal and family experience. As care practitioners, we all agree that there are not enough services and information out there for us to do our best and give evidence-based care, so we are able to give them something back. We feel that minimising emotional distress is an important part of care, as is the safety and welfare and ongoing support of people with dementia and their carers. (Lorna, Julie, Katie)

Other practitioners wrote about their 'internal values', which came from their relationships with respective grandparents:

All of us were influenced by our relationships with our grandparents, which has shaped our internal values, and our views of older people. We all made a conscious choice to work with older people and find working with people with dementia, in particular, fulfilling and worthwhile. We recognise the importance of relationship building and our specific interest in dementia care motivates us to develop, learn and practise – and hopefully influence others. (Michelle, Jo, Elizabeth, Simba)

Some practitioners identified very clearly a link between either their previous family experiences or their experiences working in dementia care and their subsequent decisions to work with persons with dementia:

We entered dementia caring by chance and common reasons for working in this area are to be able to change the way in which we nurse dementia patients. One member of the team had personal experiences of dementia with a family member, another member had poor early experiences of dementia nursing and wanted to 'do it right' this time round. The third member knew she wanted to make a career of looking after these vulnerable people very early in her nursing. (Barbara, Emily, Debbie)

In the final excerpt, from Joey, she shared her story of how she came to be working with persons with dementia. Here, the benefit of having quite a lot of autobiographical information to consider is clear in terms of understanding better her search for a role that would give her a meaningful sense of occupation:

I like to look after things. It began with books. As a child, I was horrified by people who marked their page with a folded corner or by placing their book face down. When I was a bit older, I moved on to animals. I aspired to be a vet and spent time wrapping the beloved family dog in bandages. However, work experience at the age of 15 removed my veterinary aspirations after a lady brought her dog to be euthanised. I floated through Year 11 with no aspirations, then felt I'd really found my niche when I began to study psychology at sixth form. I loved it so much I followed it on to university. We learned briefly about dementia within my course but it was somewhat overshadowed by drug addiction models, theories of anorexia and impending presentations on the nature of arsonists. My first experiences of dementia came after I'd finished my course at uni and I started working for a home care company. I met all manner of elderly people during that job but I slowly found my rotas gravitated to contain more and more 'difficult' clients – ones who wouldn't open the door, those who refused a wash, those who wouldn't allow a meal to be prepared. I found they would answer the door for me. They didn't always let me in at first but a polite tone and a friendly smile often go a long way. It turned out that over 90 per cent of my 'difficult' people had a diagnosis of dementia. I loved them. As I gained their trust they would allow me into their house, let me cook with them and help with other daily activities. Unfortunately, I had to leave that job because of financial necessity, but I looked for another job with elderly people and landed my support worker job on an orthopaedic rehab unit. Again, I found that the patients I have more rapport with, who ask if I'm on the ward, who I wonder about when I'm not at work, are the patients with dementia. They're delightful, tormented, mischievous and sometimes a real handful. But, they're always vibrant, full of spirit. Some people can only see the challenge presented by dementia patients but the relationships forged with some of these patients are my most rewarding. They really need and appreciate my care. We grow to love each other. I don't think I chose to work with dementia, I think it chose me. (Joey)

This selection of accounts from dementia care practitioners highlights some personal influences which they identify to account for how they ended up working with persons with dementia, their families and supporters. Within many is mention of the principle of wanting to care for people the way that they would want to be cared for. If knowing how to care for and support someone with dementia is related to practitioners' pre-existing experiences of dementia, then acknowledging these influences has to be important. A number of these influences are, essentially, private experiences of dementia. These include past events within families, feelings about the family member concerned and the nature of their relationships with these individuals. These private experiences also refer to practitioners' own desire to find worthwhile occupation and a role which suits their 'needs', be this to make a positive difference, to do a job that is worthwhile, or to follow through on a decision made early to work with persons with dementia.

None of this is intended to be clear cut and definitive. 'Measuring' the degree of influence is not the purpose here. It is, instead, to acknowledge these private influences. If nothing else they shine a light on what motivates some dementia care and support practitioners in their work. What is also apparent from the quotes above is that practitioners also refer to other personal experiences of dementia which are not as adequately categorised as being 'private' in origin. It is to these 'practical' experiences of dementia that attention now turns.

Practical experiences of dementia

A useful and fair way to begin a discussion of some interesting practical experiences of dementia is to return to comments made by dementia care and support practitioners during the dementia awareness study days I ran. A further observation I made, when delivering this session, was that some practitioners started to shake their heads, fold their arms and roll their eyes when discussion turned to how dementia care provision might be improved. Now, one interpretation of this kind of behaviour is to presume it implies a lack of interest in or 'negativity' towards new ideas. (Some practitioners would apologise to me privately afterwards for the 'negativity' I encountered from some of their colleagues.) However, my experience suggested this wasn't the case. In fact, this apparent rejection of different or new thinking about dementia by individuals typically highlights something I was slow to recognise.

The same message was also conveyed by practitioners when they were asked to identify the main barriers to improving dementia care and support. You may have already guessed that these barriers were usually considered to be 'time' and 'resources', followed by 'education and training'. When pressed on what they meant by 'time' and 'resources', in terms of specifying what they would be able to do better with more of both, practitioners had pretty clear ideas of how they would improve dementia care and support. These included: more time to spend getting to know, supporting and communicating with persons with dementia and with their family members or supporters; more time to engage in activities with persons with dementia; more time to read about new ideas. On the issue of 'how' this could be achieved, practitioners said that more time could only be made available if staff–person ratios were much improved, to recognise the additional time that is required to care well for someone with dementia.

Responses to requests for examples of the types of resources practitioners wanted to see often led back to staffing levels but also to the physical environment, the setting. 'Lack of stimulation' and activities were noted, as was the feeling among a significant minority that traditional hospital settings are totally inappropriate for persons with dementia. Practitioners highlighted the stark contrast between a familiar environment and the clinical setting, the lack of personally familiar objects, such as photos, and demonstrated a clear appreciation of the disorientating and confusing impacts this had on persons with dementia. There was more: the excessive, intrusive, noise, the stark lighting, the locked doors, the regimentation and the sea of unfamiliar faces, and the lack of control over the perceived poor communication practices of colleagues visiting from other settings.

As mentioned earlier, I was able to explore some of these issues further with other dementia care and support practitioners in later dementia courses that I ran. While some experiences of dementia seemed to me to be 'private' in origin, others, like those noted above, seemed to suggest a 'practical' experience of dementia, where learning about dementia comes from *doing* dementia care and support. In what follows, a series of quotes from practitioners are offered to expand on this notion of a practical experience of dementia. As is seen, this practical domain of experience offers signposts to other important sources of dementia knowledge and expertise, while sometimes also acknowledging links to the private experiences of dementia, too.

As a result of *doing* dementia care and support, some practitioners had clear ideas about what improvements were needed. It has been noted that time and resources were cited frequently but not in isolation from explanations about why this was particularly important in dementia care and what innovations they favoured. In the two examples below, the 'structure' or 'routine' of care and support was highlighted as placing limitations on what could be achieved:

> The innovations and adjustments we would like to be introduced are having more facilities with better resources, such as the specialist therapy rooms, group dining rooms, more information and staff training, enabling care to be person-centred –

individualised care, such as a relaxed structure, no set routines. (Lorna, Julie, Katie)

Our ideal is for care to be less routine- and task-orientated, for dementia care to attract the resources it deserves and for older people to count, have a voice and not be the bottom of the pile. Older age should be another chapter of a person's life, and even in institutional care, life should be 'normal', with meaningful activity and occupation, choice, responsibility, ownership and pleasure. We all feel that resources should support this, with well-trained, like-minded staff who want to make a difference in the care of people with dementia. We all recognise that good management is key to successful care. We would like to see care and services developing to meet actual needs rather than meeting targets or ticking boxes. (Michelle, Jo, Elizabeth, Simba)

Practitioners' responses on the theme of improvements to dementia care and support were rich and wide-ranging. Comments were made about better assessment processes, the involvement of persons with dementia in interview panels for staff, enhanced education and more appropriate, community-based provision:

Dementia care has moved on in recent years and a focus is now on relationship-centred nursing, involving carers and family members. What the team would like to see is a speedier and more efficient assessment process with a more relevant mini mental questionnaire, and other assessment tools to include personalised items such as photo albums and life books. At ward level, we need better interviewing processes to identify personalities and the inclusion of a person with dementia on the panel if possible. There needs to be education and information freely available for staff and family members about the different types of dementia, and flexibility with ward routines. Once a person is discharged into the community, the team would like to see provision for 'normal houses' with trained staff for supported living. Appropriate staffing levels are critical to providing relationship-centred care and we all must remember that 'memory is not everything – once their memory is gone, they are still a person!' (Barbara, Emily, Debbie)

Again, in the hospital setting, practitioners had informed opinions about what the key barriers were for all concerned and what needed to change in order that persons with dementia receive more appropriate care and support. Indication was also given about where responsibility rests for their staffing levels:

> Barriers in the acute hospital setting are many and cause distress to practitioners, patients and carers. These barriers are everything from lack of knowledge, poor environment for people with dementia, to insufficient staffing levels. The acute care setting following the 'acute phase' [of illness] is not the best place for people with dementia; therefore a speedy discharge back to their home environment is paramount to effective care. (Jayne, Jane, Michelle, Stacey)

> Needs to start at a government level in order for staffing levels to be increased to provide the positive care we should all be giving. We need to make time and get away from being task-orientated! (Alison)

One group of nurses expressed their collective desire for high-quality care, and they highlighted the importance of advocacy which, seemingly, originates in their experience of seeing dementia care and support done badly:

> We want to enrich lives, not only give basic care. It is important to us to advocate for people with dementia because we regularly see people with dementia being marginalised, ill-treated, not shown the respect that they deserve. (Michelle, Jo, Elizabeth, Simba)

There was a further discrete element of practical experience noted by a number of practitioners. While job satisfaction might be considered to be something personal or private, it seemed that, for some, the source of this satisfaction, and, specifically, the opportunity for personal development, came from their interactions with the persons with dementia with whom they worked:

> One member found it essential to have a sense of humour as a way of coping. Another member felt that the experience of caring for a person with dementia could bring out the best but also the worst in some carers. It was also felt by all that this experience could develop you personally and one member had said that this is the area for her to pursue a career in. (Barbara, Emily, Debbie)

Andrew provided a more detailed personal account of his becoming a dementia care and support practitioner. Humour was important to him, but what is perhaps most notable about his personal account is his opinion that dementia care and support work is reciprocal and, thereby, personally enriching:

> After completing a degree in film studies, I found there was no work in film and I was very poor. My mum suggested working in a nursing home as it was easy to get a job and it would tide me over until I found a proper job. I ended up really enjoying my job and after a year I began my nurse training. By this point I already knew I wanted to care for elderly patients but in my second year I had a placement on a ward specifically for acute medical patients with long-term confusion or a dementia diagnosis. Other than my year at the nursing home I had never had contact with anyone with dementia but, within a week, I knew I wanted a career in dementia care. Thankfully, at the end of my training, a job was available on the ward I had a placement on and I have been working there since. The main reason I work with people with dementia is because I laugh my ass off every day, sometimes to the point of tears – using humour as a defence mechanism can be a beautiful thing. And I can help these people that make me so happy when

they are at their most vulnerable. I love talking about my patients' pasts and also the more surreal conversations, and I love making them feel safe, valued and happy in somewhere as scary as a hospital. I feel privileged that my patients, both male and female, trust me to perform some very personal and intimate actions as a nurse and I take pride in the fact it is my own actions that create this feeling of trust. I will always groan and grumble when my alarm goes off at 5am but that's because I'm not a morning person. I never dread going to work and I always come home with a smile, and in between is surreal fun and games. (Andrew)

There are claims by two groups of practitioners that their dementia care and support practice has helped them to develop a 'special skills set', that persons with dementia contribute to their education and, as a result, to their satisfaction with their roles:

Job satisfaction – providing the best holistic care to patient or carer; personal and professional gain – a job well done! Just another skill as part of your job as a nurse – needs a set of special skills to understand [to care for] people with dementia. Not everyone has them, a lot of nurses find it difficult to understand that loss of memory and repetitive behaviour. (Jayne, Jane, Michelle, Stacey)

The team agreed that the main motivation was job satisfaction which meant different things to different members – to improve the quality of life for the person with dementia by advocating for them, protecting them, treating them with dignity and respect, realising they are individuals and unique, comforting them in times of crisis. The team felt that giving to the patient was a two-way process, gaining much satisfaction themselves. (Barbara, Emily, Debbie)

The richness and significance of this 'practical education' in dementia was suggested by one senior nurse:

The 'hands on' experience I have gained over the years in caring for people with dementia helps me to teach others and improve the quality of care they receive. (Justine)

This practical experience of dementia discussed by practitioners included an awareness of the importance of dementia education and training:

Wanting to have a positive impact on people's lives. Providing care based on how we wish to be treated ourselves. We all want to make a difference. We are also motivated by learning how to make a difference – through attending courses and using our new knowledge and ideas to empower others and facilitate change, implement best practice – after all, this is our future. It could be us and we do not want our lives to be diminished by thoughtless care! (Michelle, Jo, Elizabeth, Simba)

One group of practitioners attempted to summarise key elements in the practical experience of dementia, linking together a range of connected parts. This ranged from society and government level responses, to the significance of education and training, to the interpersonal experiences of practitioners when interacting with persons with dementia, to the skills and satisfaction that can develop with the role:

The practitioners' experience of dementia has changed in the last five years, we think, due to [the ageing] population and government reaction to this. Dementia was swept under the carpet previously but now it's so prevalent that it needs to be recognised in its own right as a debilitating disease process, with massive financial implications to the NHS and society as a whole. Practitioners' experience of dementia is bewilderment and frustration [before seeing] the light at the end of the tunnel to understanding dementia – through the introduction of education and training which sheds light on the whole complex process.

How rewarding it is now we have developed some skills to somewhere near 'caring' for people with dementia – but there is still a long way to go! (Jayne, Jane, Michelle, Stacey)

Mavis gave a frank and honest assessment of the adequacy of her dementia knowledge and how valuable she felt it would be to learn more in order to achieve her goal to improve her own practice:

I cannot really say I have a career in dementia but because I am an adult nurse working in a nursing home I found myself working with dementia patients. I don't know a lot about dementia and being on this course has made me realise that I have a lot to learn. I would like to know more about dementia because I sometimes find myself stuck/clueless when I have to deal with a dementia patient every day at work. I have attended dementia study days as a student nurse but the knowledge I have is not enough to help me in my line of work. I have developed a passion for working with dementia patients and my knowledge in dementia is improving and I hope to bring about change and perception of dementia patients in my workplace. (Mavis)

Finally, Caleb outlined some of the contours of his practical experience of dementia. In doing so, he highlighted a range of important reference points for dementia care and support practitioners, as well as the support he felt he needed to sustain him while working in his role:

I love looking after people with dementia because dementia affects mainly older adults and most of us want to live to old age and we don't know what is around the corner. Therefore, I like treating them the way I will love to be treated (golden rule). Also, I am familiar with their needs: love, comfort, companion, inclusion and occupation, and this makes my job somehow easier to plan and implement nursing care. Another reason is that I am familiar with policies, procedure and national agendas that affect people with dementia… All these help to improve practice and to relate with people with dementia, for example the National Institute for Health and Care Excellence (NICE) guideline regarding dementia care to improve service and relationships between residents and staff. I am happy with what I am doing because I bring happiness to the life of my residents as agitation and aggressive behaviour is a sign of unmet needs. To work with people with dementia you have to love older adults and make patience your watchword. I am happy caring for people with dementia because I have attended various training related to care of people with dementia in my 26 years' experience as a registered nurse and this has equipped me for the job. I also get support when I need it, for example from a consultant in old age psychiatry. Getting support is keeping me going. (Caleb)

Understanding and valuing practitioners' experiences of dementia

In summary, so far, it has been observed that dementia care and support practitioners can have a personal experience of dementia care and support, and that this has at least two dimensions, the private and the practical. Arguably, knowledge of both can aid a more meaningful understanding of dementia care practice. The contributions of those practitioners quoted above provide rich amplification of the views of other practitioners, those on the dementia awareness study days, who first got me thinking about their personal experiences of dementia. What I have since realised fully is that it was they who were the teachers in the discussion about dementia awareness, and not me.

Among them there were those who already possessed awareness of the unique, personal, drivers which motivated them in their work, and also an awareness of the uncomfortable thoughts that getting dementia aroused in them. They possessed in-depth, practical, knowledge of their settings and their politics, with ideas already formulated for what they would do better, if given the opportunity.

They had identified people outside the setting, those who set budgets, decided on the adequacy of staff–patient ratios in dementia care and support settings and, beyond that, central government funding, which set limits on what they could achieve. As a postscript to this, after acknowledging their view that external limitations, such as 'time' and 'resources', might impact on their practice, I still insisted that practitioners consider whether, in all honesty, there were things that were do-able, that could be changed by them. There were always do-able action points generated by the end of our discussions.

However, another thing stuck out for me then, as it may or may not do in your organisation, and that was the reluctance of anyone to take these matters further, to seek to let those 'in charge' know what support practitioners needed. There was a weary acceptance that 'time and resources' arguments would cut no ice. In fact, on a number of occasions I would strike a bargain with practitioners. As they committed to seek to improve their practice where they could, I committed to passing on the suggestions for improvements they had made, relating to time and resources, to the appropriate lead for dementia within the respective organisation.

Returning to those who simply shook their heads at the idea of learning something new about dementia care and support, when asked, they told me what I hadn't grasped. 'We know how to improve things, but how can we?' The penny dropped. I was thinking I was there to share ideas that practitioners might use. I realised that for a number of practitioners who were present it was as if I was encouraging them to bang their heads against a brick wall even harder. I didn't reckon on the intangibles – those aspects of care and support which dementia care practitioners have little or no leverage over. I didn't appreciate that practitioners may already be trying as hard as they thought they could to turn what they imagined really good dementia care and support could be into reality. There were reasons behind the weariness.

And it seemed as astonishing to me then as it does now that managers and dementia leads do not beat a path to the doors of those with so much collective experience and dementia intelligence, to learn from them what they *must* need to know to lead or manage dementia care services. To be fair, some organisations had 'dementia champions' or variants of this, often imprecisely defined, named dementia enthusiast or 'dementia link person' in various practice settings. However, in my experience, it was the exception rather than the rule for a coherent network of dementia intelligence-gathering to be operating within organisations and, thereby, potentially influencing strategic decision-making.

I now want to return to the detailed responses of practitioners who were asked about their personal experiences of dementia. I believe there are themes present here which suggest further examination of both the private and the practical domains of experience would be valuable. The reason for this is because of the possible understanding that might be gained about what is actually involved in *doing* relationship-centred dementia care and support. To me, there is little point in presenting an idea without then following the logic that this idea sets in train. In what follows, I outline the main themes that I feel emerge from the practitioners' accounts and explain how these are explored further in the next three chapters.

Some ways forward

The private experience of dementia has been used so far as a term to describe some of the ways that each practitioner thinks about dementia. These ways of thinking about dementia appear to originate in what has been learned about dementia and what it means, personally. This might be the impact and memory of past family experiences, sorts of formative experiences. These ways of thinking may also be traced to how each person feels when imagining what it would be like to have dementia. Further, the private experience of dementia might be a mixture of influences and decisions made in lives which have led to them choosing to work in the profession, issues perhaps of fit-to-personality and personal need. These ways of thinking are also likely to be influenced by 'public' experiences of dementia, whatever cultural or historical discourse of dementia a practitioner has grown up with in society. Ideas about the 'public' experience of dementia are not developed further here.

These are speculative ideas, based on a small sample of practitioners. Remember, however, the aim is not to generalise. Instead, what these ideas indicate is that when given the opportunity to explore personal experiences of dementia, practitioners are able to identify significant private motivations, events and feelings which, arguably, have a part to play in how they each do dementia care and support practice. This is why it is important to pause and examine the private experience of dementia in more detail and also identify some effective ways of encouraging dementia care and support practitioners to recognise and connect with their private experiences of dementia. In Chapter 5, there are some suggestions made about creative methods for going about doing this, as well as examples given of how some practitioners responded and then reflected on these methods.

The focus on practitioners' practical experiences of dementia also highlighted a number of interesting and potentially important avenues for further discussion. Again, insights about these forms of learning about dementia came from practitioners themselves. The two themes identified from what the practitioners had to say included one which could be called 'practical expertise', the result of practical experience. A number of comments that were made under this theme related to individual and collective expertise about the realities of dementia care and support practice. These could be a source of satisfaction or of frustration and were described as being relevant not only to them but also to persons with dementia and their family members and supporters. Further, some practitioners identified barriers to improvement in practice and also suggested where responsibility for this rests.

Acknowledgement of practice expertise suggests the existence of rich and credible sources of information about what actually goes on in dementia care and support services, known to individual practitioners and to those within their immediate practice communities. In Chapter 6, this idea of dementia communities of practice is examined in more detail, looking at the potential role of the individual dementia care and support practitioner to maximise their membership of the communities of practice available to them. To imagine this more positively, the notion of the 'lead participant' in relationship-centred dementia care and support is refined. This is done by recognising more explicitly the passion for high-quality services which characterises the accounts provided by practitioners in this chapter. Alison Gordon's notion of the 'dementia passionista' is presented here to provoke discussion, as are Natasha Wilson's ideas about a 'dementia tribe' (see Chapter 6).

There is a second theme which embraces a number of the points made by practitioners in relation to their practical experiences of dementia. This is more a status than it is a conventional theme. In the accounts given above there were references made to the important role that education plays in supporting practitioners to understand dementia and guide practice. Some of this education was peer education. However, it is a focus on the other, formal types of education and training that I seek to develop further. In addition, some practitioners referred to the importance of policy, of maintaining an understanding of dementia policy, such as the guidance produced by the National Institute for Health and Care Excellence (2020a).

What is argued here is that dementia care and support practitioners, whether they realise it or not, warrant status as members of these 'dementia standards' communities, too. Dementia standards communities include those that produce dementia guidance and quality standards for services (e.g. National Institute for Health and Care Excellence, 2018, 2019) and those that produce recommendations for dementia education (e.g. Skills for Health, Skills for Care and Health Education England, 2015, 2018). It follows that if dementia care and support practitioners have accumulated experience and expertise in the practical delivery of care and support services, then it is worth exploring the ways in which practitioners engage with their dementia standards communities and, also, how those standards communities demonstrate that they value practitioner expertise. These matters are discussed further in Chapter 7.

Summary

This chapter turned the spotlight on dementia care practitioners' personal experiences of dementia. It was argued that these perspectives are under-appreciated but essential to explore in a relationship-centred approach to dementia care and support. A focus on these perspectives suggested two dimensions which could be significant to better understanding what actually happens in dementia care and support practice. These are practitioners' private and practical experiences of dementia. A focus on the private experiences of dementia raises awareness of the existence of motivational factors, fears and the effects of what can be described as their emotional labour. A case was made for dementia care and support practitioners to be given greater opportunity to reflect on and consider their personal experiences of dementia and the impacts these might have on their practice.

With this focus on the practical experiences of dementia it was shown that care practitioners have high levels of aspiration for service quality. They also possess knowledge about and frustrations with some of the intangible barriers they see as impeding service improvement. The intelligence that dementia care and support practitioners possess was argued to provide vital insights, should organisations and their decision-makers choose to value and then access them. While dementia care practitioners are lead participants, and have associated responsibilities in each episode of care and support, responsibility for improvements to dementia care and support is not and cannot be theirs alone. It was argued that practitioners belong to a number of significant communities of dementia practice about which questions arise as to how and in what ways their expertise is valued.

on and consider their practical experiences of dementia and the impact these might have on their practice.

With this focus on the practical experiences of dementia it was shown that care practitioners have high levels of aspiration for service quality. They also possess knowledge about and frustrations with some of the intangible barriers they see as impeding service improvement. The intelligence that dementia care and support practitioners possess was argued to provide vital insights, should organisations and their decision-makers choose to value and then access them. While dementia care practitioners are lead participants and have associated responsibilities in each episode of care and support, responsibility for improvements to dementia's care and support is not and cannot be theirs alone. It was argued that practitioners belong to a number of significant communities of dementia practice about which questions are as to how and in what ways their expertise is valued.

CHAPTER 5

Creative Approaches to Exploring Practitioners' Private Experiences of Dementia

In this chapter, there is an exploration of how engaging in creative, reflective activities might help you to develop a clearer appreciation of your own attitudes towards dementia, persons with dementia and family members and supporters. Building on Chapter 4, it is suggested that dementia care and support practitioners possess their own private experiences of dementia – sources of knowledge that are specific to each individual but which exclude practical experience that is learned by doing the job. This form of knowledge is, by definition, private and hidden. It is hidden – not in the sense that anyone deliberately hides it – but in the sense of it not being obvious or available to anyone else to know, unless you choose to share it. And, it isn't something adequately described as simply 'knowledge', like books on a library shelf. In some of the accounts given by practitioners in the previous chapter, it is fairly obvious that there can be strong emotions associated with some of these experiences. These emotions, linked to private experiences, might hold sway in the decisions and actions practitioners take.

Whether it is to your taste or not I have tried to be open in my introduction to this book and throughout about what I feel has influenced my own thinking: the people, the ideas, and how these have influenced the approach to dementia care and support that I advocate. There are likely to be other influences which I am unaware of, too. My point is that I feel it is helpful to be candid about these known influences in order that I can understand better the bases of my ideas and so can anyone else who might read about them. If you can understand where you are 'coming from' in dementia care and support, you can explain this to others – and then others have what they need to contribute their perspective, discuss, debate and disagree. So why do you, a dementia care practitioner, approach your work in care and support the way you do?

This is a central concern of this chapter. It relates tangentially to a wider issue about dementia in society, that of 'dementia awareness'. I have to be honest and say I find this notion a bit confusing. The premise is that among us all in society there are those with beliefs and ideas about dementia that propagate and perpetuate negative, unhelpful, stereotypes. This much I get. However, at what point can it be claimed that dementia awareness has improved? What is it that is being measured? What is the baseline, the starting point? Who is measuring this? I mention this because one of the questions I have had in my mind when delivering dementia awareness sessions to care practitioners is in relation to what individuals already know about dementia from their personal experiences. Alongside private and practical experiences of dementia we might also add this somewhat nebulous 'public' experience of dementia.

Care practitioners are, of course, members of their societies, subject to cultural and historical influences that make up all of our 'dementia baggage' which, in turn, sticks to or contaminates the term 'dementia'. It should be noted here that not everyone shares what might be considered to be the same cultural and historical influences with regards to 'dementia', given that the UK is a multi-ethnic community and that, for some people, the term 'dementia' is not commonly used and, when translated, can create significant stigma (All-Party Parliamentary Group on Dementia, 2013, Chapter 6; Jeraj and Butt, 2018). Forgive me for swerving this important element of complexity but it is worthy of far greater scrutiny than I can afford it here. Instead, I make a point which probably applies to all, and that is, enmeshed within the sorts of personal experiences discussed previously, there is also, presumably, the influences which improved dementia awareness is supposed to counteract or nullify. Therefore, it is sensible to suggest that care practitioners' personal experiences of and, therefore, attitudes towards dementia need to be viewed as some combination of their private experiences, practical experiences and 'cultural baggage' – their public experience.

Where one stops and others begin is not important here and, in any case, it would be a futile task to attempt to separate these threads. The point is simply to remember that dementia care practitioners are not a special type of person, immune to their own historical and cultural dementia narratives. Expecting practitioners to think only positive things about dementia because of their specialist role in care and support is unrealistic and unhelpful. From this point, I will say no more about the public experiences of dementia, having pointed out it is likely to contribute to a practitioner's overall personal experiences of dementia.

Recognising that dementia care and support practitioners have their own private experiences of dementia is one thing. Finding ways to explore these in productive and safe ways is another. I found that in short education or training sessions it was difficult to get to a point whereby practitioners felt comfortable revealing their feelings about dementia. And, if this did happen, there was insufficient time to consider how knowing more, through them reflecting on their private experiences, might lead to improvements in dementia care and support. At the time, I had developed an interest in the creative arts in dementia and had begun coordinating the South Yorkshire Dementia Creative Arts Exhibition (Reid, 2014). As well as being an attempt to bring together the local dementia community, the annual event was intended to offer those affected by dementia, including dementia care practitioners, an opportunity to showcase their skills and talents.

As a result of this experience, I began to think more about the potential of creative expression to open up a dialogue about the kinds of personal meanings held by dementia care practitioners. Below, I provide more information about how I sought to do this, as well as some of the outcomes of this approach, along with feedback from practitioners who participated. Before I do this, I would like to ask you to do what I have asked many practitioners, students and colleagues to do when I have begun a session on dementia. This requires you to avoid the temptation to read on after I set you a short task. If you're up for it, please now get yourself a piece of paper and a pen or pencil. You'll need a quiet space where you won't be interrupted to do this, and it'll take five to ten minutes.

What I am going to ask you to do involves reflecting a little on your thoughts about dementia, and so, as I would say to you in person, please be aware that thinking about dementia can be emotional, depending on your life experiences, and do not undertake this task if you suspect it might be very upsetting.

Okay. This is the task. I would like you to think about 'dementia'. Think about this word and what it conjures up for you in your mind. Maybe write it down at the top of your blank sheet of paper. What does it make you think of? How does it make you feel? There are no right or wrong answers. Allow yourself to think until you have something in mind. Then, please use your pen or pencil to draw 'dementia', that is, what you are thinking about, what dementia means to you. The only rule is that you are not allowed to use any words in your drawing. Please start when you are ready and read on when you are finished.

While people were drawing or scratching their heads or looking at me shaking their heads (again) with bemusement or even barely concealed hatred, I would walk around and, with anticipation, glance down at the kinds of images that were being produced. To me, this was very exciting, while to those in the room it was, well, an unusual request, to say the least. Who goes to a dementia training session expecting to draw? What kind of image did you produce? In fact, if you want, you can email the image to me, anonymously if you prefer (daredementia@gmail.com). I'd be interested to see it and will reply to anyone who does this.

When everyone had finished I then invited each person to show the rest of the group what they had drawn, and explain the reasoning behind it. I have to say that like any discussion of something which may be of such personal significance, this kind of exercise was sometimes upsetting for some. I have seen people become very emotional when trying to explain their drawings, including dementia care practitioners.

I found that in the vast majority of cases, participants wanted to speak about what they produced. In doing so, individuals began to reveal feelings and thoughts about dementia that would not have been accessible had they instead been asked to think and then write, rather than draw. Also, the rule about not using words (not always followed) prompted the use of imagery, of scenarios, of objects – forms of visual metaphor, perhaps. Now, before I am accused of pretending to be some kind of expert skilled in the interpretation of visual metaphor, or a psychologist who might comment in an informed way on what these images might reveal about a person's thought processes, I'm not. I'm simply curious about ways of accessing how practitioners and others think about dementia. To me, these drawings are starting points for further, deeper discussions about our personal views and perspectives on dementia. 'Dementia' is a single word but, clearly, has many personal interpretations.

For the record, there were a number of recurrent themes among the hundreds of drawings that I have seen in response to setting this task. If you haven't yet completed the task and want to know how yours might fit in – if at all – with the kinds of images others have produced, this is your last chance to go back and do this. Okay, common themes included the following: depictions of a signpost with question marks above it; paths leading off in meandering ways into a distant horizon; individuals with confused expressions with question marks over their heads; family members separated from their loved ones, either by the use of space to indicate this or zig zag lines; people with their memories disappearing; people incarcerated in institutions or cut off from loved ones outside; walls and various barriers between people and 'normal life'; and a focus on brains – fracturing, emptying or decaying.

Rarely was there present any imagery which might be interpreted as 'positive'. There were some, such as when loved ones held hands with or were embraced by the person depicted with dementia, or where the person with dementia wore a smile. In the vast majority of drawings, the person with dementia was old and infirm (i.e. walking sticks, frames, sitting in high-backed chairs, heavily lined faces) and isolated and confused. These kinds of insights are not intended to be viewed as definitive, to be the last word on how someone might think about dementia. They can, however, be indicative and a point for discussion about dementia and what it means to practitioners, about dementia knowledge, stereotypes and practical obstacles for those affected by dementia. Approached in this way, training and education can then shape to fit the issues, topics and feelings that originate with practitioners, making it inherently personal.

As an extension of this idea that creativity can offer ways into greater self-awareness of attitudes and beliefs about dementia, I have previously included a one-day session on a ten-session dementia education course. Working with a qualified art therapist (Sally Weston), who led and structured the sessions (I did not participate), the idea was for practitioners to explore personal meanings of dementia while gaining a taste of the rationale and methods of art therapy. Sally explains her approach below. This is followed by some examples of artwork which practitioners produced during these sessions, and feedback from some on their experiences of taking part.

ART THERAPY SESSIONS, BY SALLY WESTON

Art therapy offers opportunity for self-expression using art media within a therapeutic relationship. It is offered to people who are facing change or loss, have experienced trauma or are in mental or emotional distress. It is available on the NHS and generally offered to people for whom verbal expression is difficult or who have complex issues that cannot be easily put into words. Art therapists work with people with long-standing mental health problems, with learning difficulties, people in palliative care, children in the mental health teams and in schools, with brain injury including stroke, dementia and other neurological conditions. It is accessible and very client-centred – the therapist follows where the client and their creative processes or imagination lead them!

When approached by David to offer an introduction to art therapy to the students on the course, I was keen to ensure that students experienced something of the power of the process for themselves. We all understand the world through our senses and through play before we develop language. These symbolic, metaphoric and tactile ways of understanding the world and ourselves, far from being childish, can be intensely meaningful in adult life too. It can be painful or extremely pleasurable to make something. The process can take us through a progression of different thoughts and feelings as we work. It can shift difficulties or it can be an expression – a celebration, for example, of something important to us. These processes are equally accessible to people whose verbal reasoning is challenged.

The sessions begin with a brief introduction to art therapy as a particular way of working, its psychodynamic roots and the frameworks and boundaries art therapists employ to make their work safe and effective. We also look at the development in this country and the ways it might help people with dementia. I give a brief talk about my work and present a case study looking at the artwork of a woman with severe short-term memory problems.

The main part of the day, however, is the experiential session. I have developed workshops over the years working with other staff in the NHS. With the dementia care and support practitioners, I introduce art therapy by asking participants to pick up a paintbrush, piece of clay or some collage materials to have a go at making something. They are asked to take note of the thoughts and feelings that they experience and then we look together at what has been made and share with others something about this process.

While the session cannot be seen as therapy, it can give a flavour of the process. My hope is always that participants can feel safe enough to work on something and get in touch with something significant and meaningful to them. This may be having the opportunity to make space, to feel calm and reflective in a busy day, or it might be being able to work on some tricky issue. Participants need to feel safe enough to do this, and a paradoxical aspect of art-making in an art therapy group is that while the work is done it can also be seen by all. It is made individually, often in a quiet, intense, atmosphere where quite private thoughts can be pursued.

In art therapy, people are generally asked if they can reflect on their work, but there is no obligation to speak. The work can speak for itself or not be brought into the group. Art therapy has been influenced by psychodynamic thinking and a belief in the power of the unconscious. Art therapists in England are quite heavily influenced by a Jungian thinking on the unconscious – that images, and the arts, are expressions of the unconscious and means of seeking health and resolution.

Care needs to be taken in responding to images made. Their meaning is only truly known to the person who made them, although this may not be entirely on a conscious level. The best response is often to let the pictures speak for themselves. When students are invited to experiment with an art material of their choice, in any group of students, reactions to this idea will vary and I try to ensure that everyone feels they can join in. I check out how people are feeling about the session. Generally, there is a range of feelings at the beginning of the day, from confidence and eager anticipation, to dread! I introduce the art materials and offer help to anyone who wants to know about the materials or gets stuck in starting. People are urged to forget about the finished product but to get involved in the process. Confidentiality and the reassurance that the work is not assessed or even seen by anyone outside the group are important in ensuring that people can get started. In the discussion that follows, I usually make the point that the range of experience in the group is not unlike any group of people embarking on art therapy.

The second art-making session is an opportunity to reflect on dementia. This can be reflection using the art materials or a situation or person at work that is on their minds, or an aspect of the course they would like to think about. However, if they have something that has been stirred up from the earlier session that they would like to pursue, they can work on that. This session can lead to wider-ranging discussions on the experience of art-making and on the need for time for reflection as well as action in the working day – and what impact this might have on the people with whom we work and the services we offer.

An important aspect of the way that I and many others practise art therapy is that it is non-directive. The object is to allow clients to find and explore their own issues in their own time and to find what art media best suits this expression. This does not mean that at the beginning help isn't given in getting started. The wide range of choice is aimed to make sure that people can pursue what is important to them at that time. When working with people who may not be able to let you know what is going on in their minds, respecting that, even though you may not understand, what the person is doing is meaningful and makes sense to them is important. Of course, sharing the experience of looking at a picture together does not need words.

I make the point that some people like to be led by the process of making – to assemble some art or collage materials and see what happens. Others prefer to start from a specific theme or idea. This is how different artists work and there is no right or wrong. In the course of the workshop, I make sure there is opportunity for both ways of working. In the course of the day, people can learn about themselves but also from how others work and what they say.

The art therapist needs to be prepared to stay with difficult feelings such as loss, grief and anger, as well as affirm positive feelings, celebrations and memories. Feelings can be expressed in the art as well as to the therapist. These are the difficult feelings that art therapists are trained to work with and, hopefully, they can help alleviate some of that distress. I hope the session shows that while non-art therapists would not be expected to actively work with these issues, they can still acknowledge the wide range of feelings that come up and feel more confident in working with clients creatively. The students I have worked with have entered into the art therapy sessions with courage and honesty.

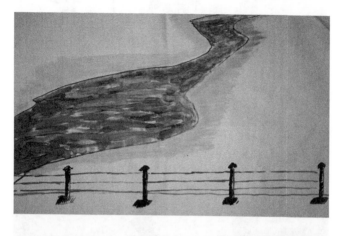

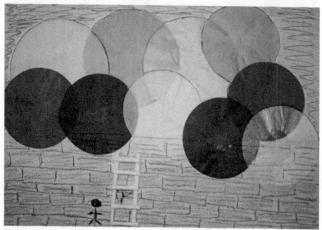

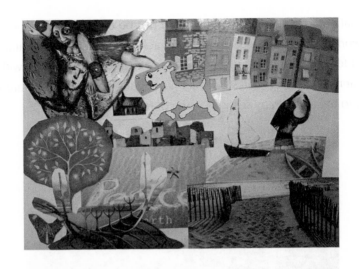

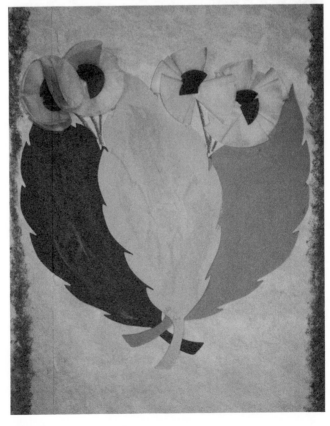

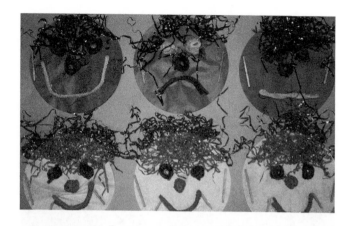

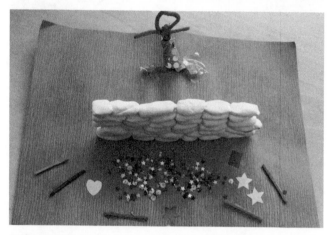

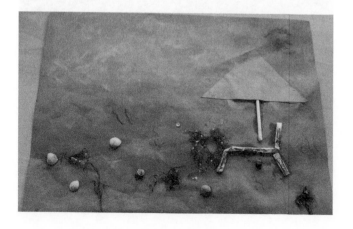

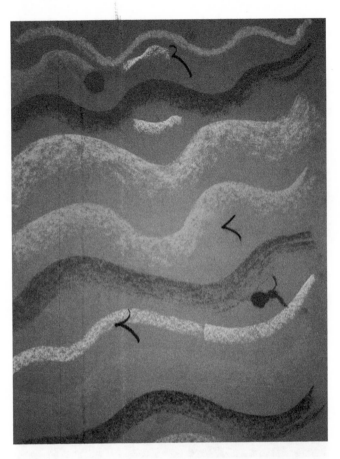

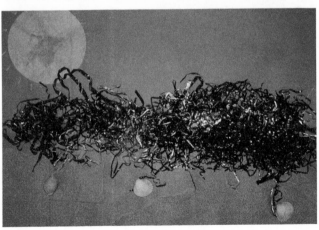

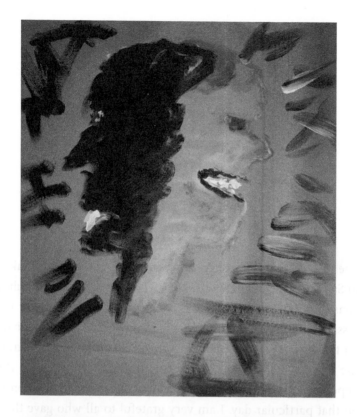

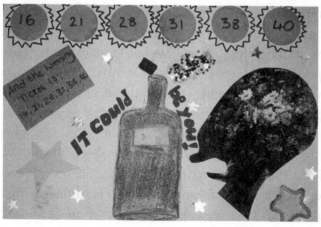

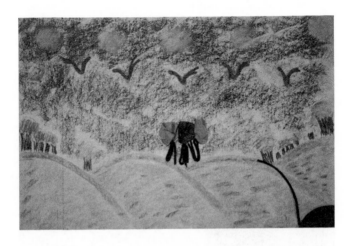

The images reproduced here are from creative work undertaken in Sally's art therapy sessions. They were not intended for public consumption and scrutiny. I asked some practitioners after the sessions if I could photograph and use images of their creativity for the purpose that they are presented here – that is, to illustrate the sorts of images and ideas they produced when given the opportunity to reflect on their personal feelings about dementia on that particular day. I am very grateful to all who gave their permission because what it does, this sharing, is help open up discussion about the private experiences of dementia, practitioner to practitioner. By sharing like this, these dementia care and support practitioners are, I hope, contributing to new learning about dementia, inspiring others in the wider dementia care and support practitioner community to spark new peer learning.

Like the description of my 'drawing dementia' exercise that preceded them, the selection of images is intended to be indicative. There is nothing definitive to conclude about the private experiences of dementia care and support practitioners. To do so would be to fall into the same trap that awaits those who use the terms 'people with dementia' or 'carers' to force unwarranted and unhelpful generalisations about the diverse experiences of groups of people. This is no justification or desire to suggest that any of the images or ideas presented are your experience, your imagining of dementia. Sharing these images is only to demonstrate something of what creative art offers practitioners – and everyone – as a means by which to communicate things that words cannot always fully capture. Here is some feedback from practitioners on their experiences of taking part in the art therapy sessions:

As a creative person anyway I was very enthusiastic about the art therapy session and I have to say I enjoyed it immensely! When I saw all the different materials, paints, chalks and so on, I felt like a child in a sweet shop. After I had collected the materials I set to work and made a picture of a bright yellow daisy-like flower, very colourful with a red border! The whole exercise reminded me of my old school days; you could have heard a pin drop in that room, the whole group sat there in a disciplined-like way. We must have all been pouring out our thoughts and feelings while producing those pictures because talking about them afterwards revealed positive and negative comments. It was all positive for me, I felt happy while I was doing my picture, and I was happy with the end result. (Rose)

After initial trepidation, I got to admit really enjoyed this session, found it very calming and effective. (Sharon)

I believe art therapy plays a huge part when undertaking therapeutic activities. I felt some people in the group felt a little nervous prior to 'having a go'. Because I've undertaken this before I knew what was expected, and you don't have to be an artist in any shape or form. It's about interaction and, foremost, communication. I really enjoyed the session! (John Paul)

The art therapy session was something I was quite apprehensive about as art is not one of my strengths. We were given a vast range of art materials to complete two pictures, the first being anything that depicted a place where I was happy and content and the second one was to demonstrate how a patient with dementia may feel. After a lot of deliberation, I decided to use collage for both my pictures. My first was a collage of a beach and deep blue sea with shells on the beach. While compiling the picture we talked among ourselves about what we were making and why. Using the glue to stick pieces of material to the paper reminded me of my school days. I used to put the glue all over my fingers and spend the rest of the day picking it off. I was not surprised to hear that I was not the only one who used to do this! After we had all completed our first picture we sat as a group and discussed them. A lot of us had used holidays as our theme. (Lynn)

I can also see that for some people the art might be what is needed but, speaking personally, I actually found it quite threatening, if that's the right word. It took me straight back to the horrors of art at school. It has made me think though that perhaps we should re-write the list of things we would want people to know about us because for me art is a definite no! Thanks for being there, Sue! I'm not sure what it was, I found the atmosphere in the room very intense, which then led on to the feeling of 'pressure' to produce some art. Personally, I find colouring relaxing/therapeutic, but having to produce a picture from a blank canvas is very stressful. I'm sorry this sounds very negative, doesn't it? I can see that for some people it would be a good thing, but it has also shown me that what would be a good form of therapy for one person would be a total disaster for another, which I suppose leads me back to knowing more about the backgrounds of the people who I care for. (Jessica)

For my second picture, I drew a brick wall with chalk and then stuck a ladder made from straws onto the wall with a matchstick man at the bottom, this being the person with dementia. On the other side of the wall I used different brightly coloured tissue paper and coloured paper to create a bright and cheerful theme that the person with dementia was trying to reach. Again, we discussed our pictures as a group. Although the pictures were different in style, they all had the same theme: the person with dementia being in a dark place and a bright coloured area that they were trying to reach. After participating in the art therapy session, I can appreciate how this would benefit people with dementia to express their feelings. It is not just the fact that they are creating a picture but that they are socialising with others. (Lynn)

I found the art session the most difficult session of the whole course, if I am being truly honest, because I found it the most challenging on an emotional level. This is because I was not expecting it to have such a powerful impact on me personally. I had not fully realised how art can unleash deep feelings within the individual. In the first exercise, after initially trying to plan to paint something which may have been deemed appropriate or relevant by the rest of the group and the art therapist so that I would not lose face, I began just to let go of my initial anxieties and allow myself to open up to what was going on inside me on a deeper level. I found that [as] I began to paint in a more spontaneous and less contrived way, the exercise became less an onerous task and more something personal and private to me. I found that the exercise brought to my consciousness aspects I had clearly sought to repress and deny. I had sad and depressive thoughts in my subconscious which I had been unwilling to acknowledge openly. Once I became aware of this, I felt a lightening of feeling – the hidden had become visible and I felt an instant relief. This experience then opened up a way for me to begin to deal with these feelings of sadness and darkness in a positive way. Thus, the exercise was clearly therapeutic for me – it gave me a valuable insight into something important I had to deal with. After the session had ended I was able to start to do this. It thus allowed me to see how powerful art could be and how useful if it could be used in a practical way. It gave me a greater respect for its therapeutic use. It made me want to explore more how art could be used in my workplace for the benefit of the residents I work with. (John)

Quite surprised how much I enjoyed it as it was one session I felt a little nervy about. I found it interesting how people interpreted pieces of work that others had produced, also the expressive pieces of E and S, makes you view things in a totally different light. (Vivienne)

My question to you, as someone who is lead participant in interactions with persons with dementia, family members and supporters, is how, if at all, do your private experiences of dementia influence your work? Feedback from care practitioners who participated in these art therapy day-long sessions gives some indication of where this influence might be located, where it might explain actions – the action of doing dementia care and support. For example, could private experience in some way set limits on what you do, inhibiting the extent to which you are comfortable interacting with persons with dementia, perhaps in what you would be confident to discuss? At the other extreme, does your private experience serve to propel you into meaningful interaction, triggering a mindset, attitude and body language which are open, receptive and engaged?

By opening up about the possible significance of private experiences of dementia to practitioners' interactions with persons with dementia, there is not only the possibility created for sharing and for mutual learning with colleagues, but also, importantly, a step away from blaming 'problems' in communication on persons with dementia and considering the origins of some difficulties as, instead, residing with practitioners. This honest and fair reappraisal can only occur if practitioners are given credit for possessing their own subjective experiences of dementia and afforded the appropriate time, methods, reflective space and blame-free environment in which to do this.

A second approach I have used to invite dementia care and support practitioners to discuss their private experiences of dementia is through the use of music. Like the art therapy sessions, these day-long events were inspired by practitioners' ideas. While the art-based sessions seem a useful means by which to explore private meanings of dementia, the music sessions were offered as a route to explore further this idea of 'caring for someone in the way I would like to be cared for'. Until writing this now, I've never decided fully what it was I was hoping to achieve. However, as push has come to shove I feel the main aim was to encourage dementia care and support practitioners to view themselves as possessing unique biographies or lives as do, of course, the persons with dementia with whom they interact. In short, if it is true that some imagine they are offering care and support to 'themselves', what is it about themselves that it is significant for others to know?

The musical element is a vehicle for exploring these significant matters, and I outline the specific task below. Before I do so, I want to share a further way that I have sought to encourage dementia care and support practitioners to acknowledge the uniqueness of their personal biographies. This didn't involve music but the oft-dreaded 'role play'. In an education or training session, I have asked dementia care and support practitioners to imagine that they live in a care home, that they have dementia and that they experience communication impairments. The lead into this exercise was typically preceded by a collective acknowledgement that, statistically speaking, it was likely that six or seven among the 20 or so practitioners present would develop a form of dementia if everyone lived to 80 years of age.

So, they are all living in a care home (stay with me on this!) and they are lucky, because some years ago in a dementia awareness training session they were asked to prepare some information for a care practitioner who would be offering them care and support in the home. I'd explain that this is what we were doing right now, preparing that information. The task I set was to ask practitioners to write down three things that they thought this member of staff would need to know about them, in order to treat them the way they would want to be treated. It is, admittedly, a clumsily worded task. However, the idea is that these three 'facts' would appear on a bullet-point list which the dementia care and support practitioner would read and, for the sake of argument, would act on in good faith. As you read this you may wish to pause and write down three things about you that you might like a dementia care practitioner to know about you, in those circumstances.

I was asked once afterwards by a participant if I could post their list to them, in the future, if they got dementia. I have to say I spent too long considering the temporal-spatial logistics of this particular request! But, the responses participants came up with included statements such as: 'Treat me with respect', 'Make sure that I'm clean', 'I was a nurse', 'Please keep my teeth clean', 'I like tea, intravenously, and I hate coffee – don't give me coffee!', 'I prefer a shower every day and not a bath', 'I must have a glass of red wine/beer/vodka every evening', 'I want to be outside in the fresh air because I loved walking my dog'.

There was such a variety of points, and we shared lots of fun as well as earnest discussion – and special pleading from some for four points rather than three (answer: no, only three). Away from the fun, the aim was for dementia care and support practitioners to 'feel' a little of the pressure to get this right, for them to see in themselves and in persons with dementia, and their possible future selves, their non-negotiable, vital, personal characteristics, preferences and needs. The reliance on others was plain to see, as was the sense that, should they not have these aspects of themselves respected, they were likely to notice this and communicate their dissatisfaction through their behaviour. I asked them whether their behaviour might be viewed as 'challenging'; thereby a further connection was made with how persons with dementia might become labelled as exhibiting 'challenging behaviour' for rejecting inappropriate or impersonal forms of care and support.

Back to the music. Dementia care and support practitioners were asked, the week before the session, to choose a piece of music that they would hate to think they would never hear again. This is another awkwardly phrased task but it was, in my defence, a more open request than being asked for your favourite piece of music or a significant piece of music. In any case, participants were asked to send a digital copy of the piece of music or a hyperlink to where it could be accessed online or, old school, bring with them a CD the following week. In this way, we were able to create a 'playlist' for the group and, with apologies every time, I brought some Phil Collins so I could participate as well. And then, in the teaching room, we listened to music all day, much to the bewilderment and sometimes irritation of others in the adjoining rooms.

The order in which each piece of music was played was determined on the day. If there was reluctance among the group about who was going to start, then I would volunteer. After each person's music was played, he or she was invited, but was not obliged, to explain a little about the significance of their piece of music. It was in these explanations that practitioners' lives opened up. Memories were shared, people and places illuminated, spiritual beliefs revealed, key moments in lives described and the accompanying emotions, then and now, made real. It was an honour to be able to listen to these personal accounts, and one of the defining qualities of these sessions was the respect that practitioners showed one another. What was said was treated confidentially, and while this was, rightly, flagged at the start of the session, it was evident throughout that everyone appreciated the sensitivity with which such sharing should be approached.

The feedback from participants indicates how they valued this particular opportunity:

> I really enjoyed this morning, hearing everyone's music, even though I found it quite emotional. I feel really comfortable with our group so it felt safe. (Sue)

> The music therapy class involved bringing to class a piece of music I enjoyed listening to and would hate never to hear again. For me, the session was quite emotional. It brought back memories of both good and bad times I have had within my life. My piece of music was titled 'No Matter What' by Boyzone. Its meaning for me is that no matter what life throws at you, there is always someone there to help get you through the rough and smooth. The session highlighted the many different tastes people have in music and what it means to them. It also demonstrated how music allows people with dementia to communicate their feelings. I have used music therapy since the session with some of our patients who have a diagnosis of dementia to help reduce their agitation, with amazing results. (Lynn)

> I thought it was a very enjoyable session, that made the point that we are all different and all enjoy different types of music, as will our patients. It reinforces the point that you cannot sit a group of people in a room together and play one kind of music, expecting everyone to enjoy it – people with dementia very much included. (Theresa)

> What an enjoyable day it was today. I especially enjoyed listening to E's music. I feel that listening to everyone's accounts of their special music gave me more of an insight into each other and our personalities. It's made me realise I need to start listening to my music more often and maybe get the kids to listen to theirs

via their iPods in their rooms instead of subjecting me and my partner to their choices of music. Lol. This could be an example of staff subjecting people with dementia to their choice of music instead of listening to what the person with dementia would like to listen to. (Julie)

The music was brilliant, emotional I know, but I could have happily done that all day, and at work we have started trying with various pieces of music in our unit with, so far (early days I know), quite a positive, calming effect. (Jessica)

The music session for me was a mixture of emotions. My music choice made me feel proud, sad and happy. Bringing back those memories made me think how lucky I am to have had such a wonderful caring mother and how I miss her so much. It was also interesting to hear the music choices of the rest of the group which for some were positive, happy memories and for others negative, sad times. Looking back now, I think that although the group had only recently met and didn't know each other very well, listening to their music and what it meant to them showed an insight into their lives. All in all, the music session was a warming experience. (Rose)

To me, the use of carefully chosen music to evoke events in private lives was particularly powerful. Their music offered a motorway to places, times, values, people, all conjured, brought to life and felt. The richness of each practitioner's life was suggested in these brief invitations. While these typically had nothing whatsoever to do with dementia, the act of opening up, and the special way music does this, offers another creative way to think about dementia care and support.

I believe music does this by encouraging you to recognise the precious and unique nature of your own and colleagues' personal biographies. When seeking to care for and support someone in the way you would like to be cared for and supported yourself, there is consequently a greater, richer imagining of the person with dementia in front of you. This originates in an enhanced appreciation of your own lived experiences, the significance of things, of memories, and the value of this appreciation to dementia care and support practice. The ongoing significance of music to persons with dementia has been recognised for some time (see e.g. the provision of professional musicians in care homes by Lost Chord, 2020), and bespoke approaches, similar to the one I used with dementia care and support practitioners, have been developed for persons with dementia and their families and supporters (e.g. Playlist for Life, 2019).

Summary

The aim of this chapter has been to focus on the private experiences of dementia care and support practitioners. It has been argued that such private meanings can go unrecognised but can play an important role in influencing why and how dementia care and support practitioners *do* dementia care and support. Invisible, intangible yet influential, a few methods from the arts have been described which could offer practitioners ways to explore these meanings. Using drawing and art therapy methods and approaches can help practitioners to gain a greater appreciation of how they feel about dementia which then represent starting points for further discussions of how this might translate into or influence their practice, and their ability to interact with persons with dementia, their family members and supporters.

Choosing music with personal significance also offers dementia care and support practitioners novel means by which to develop an appreciation of the power of music to deliver, fast, memories that by extension they would hate to think they would lose. By recognising in themselves the precariousness of personal biography, when they seek to care for or support someone in the way they would like to be cared for, there is a greater rather than lesser imagining of the person (with dementia) in front of them.

In the next chapter, attention turns from the private and public experiences of dementia to the practical experiences of dementia. With an argument for extending the idea of the 'lead participant' to account for the passion many dementia care and support practitioners have for their roles, this is a focus on the knowledge, learning and potential of working as a dementia care practitioner within a number of communities of practice.

CHAPTER 6

Engaging with your Dementia Communities of Practice

The identification of a practical domain to care and support practitioners' experiences of dementia is not to point out anything particularly novel. However, focusing on practitioners' practical experiences of dementia provides a space to discuss and consider practical 'expertise' gained through doing dementia care and support, as opposed to the private and, to a lesser extent, public experiences of dementia which have been topics of discussion in the previous two chapters. The distinction between private, public and practical domains is artificial when it comes to explaining what practitioners do in practice, which will be a unique combination of all three influences. The distinction, as noted before, is simply to make it easier to discuss different types of influence which might shape practitioners' dementia care and support practice.

The practical domain of experience takes in the knowledge, skills and opportunities that dementia care and support practitioners have as a result of working alongside persons with dementia, family members and supporters and, importantly, their practice colleagues in particular settings. The discussion that follows makes some assumptions to simplify matters further. First, dementia care practitioners are viewed as working in a single care or support setting. Second, as a consequence, practitioners are assumed to have a team of colleagues with whom they work in that setting. Third, no detailed attention is paid to the expertise which practitioners might have gained in other settings prior to the one they now work in. Fourth, it is assumed that those delivering frontline dementia care and support do not manage the overall care or support service.

The value of pointing out these limitations at the start may become obvious as you read on. Nonetheless, it is hoped that the ideas presented here are of some value to all dementia care and support practitioners. In the previous two chapters, a number of arguments have been made for taking more seriously the experiences of dementia care and support practitioners. These are restated concisely in an attempt to show more clearly the links I am trying to make in proposing a critical, relationship-centred approach to dementia care and support. This approach places the practitioner in a unique and influential position in episodes of dementia care and support. Both the person with dementia and the family member or supporter are considered to have their own unique experiences of life, lived with dementia. They are the experts in their experiences and, as *lead participant* in these communication relationships, the practitioner has responsibility to learn about their expertise, then draw on this proactively in the care or support which they offer. Learning and acting on what is learned are key activities.

It has also been suggested that each dementia care and support practitioner has their own experiences of dementia which may influence how they do their work. Rather than accepting, as often seems the case, that those working in dementia care only require education or training – with this 'expertise' being conveyed in a so-called 'top-down' direction – it is argued that a 'down-up' direction for sharing expertise is required. Practitioners have expert knowledge and skills which have been undervalued and under-utilised. Further, dementia care and support practitioners have been shown to have private experiences of dementia which, one way or another, probably exert some influence over the ways they do dementia care and support. This might be the memory of a loved one fuelling their motivation, ideas about what they would want if it was them who had dementia shaping their response to someone they are supporting, or perhaps the fear associated with developing dementia themselves inhibiting their interactions with persons with dementia.

It has been noted, too, that the quality of dementia care and support in any setting cannot and should not be the sole responsibility of any one practitioner. This is an appropriate place to begin exploring the practical domain in the experiences of dementia care and support practitioners. One of the consistent failings of ideas about improving dementia care is, in my view, the absence of any meaningful consideration of the working context within which dementia care practice and support is offered. It simply cannot be the case that improvements to dementia care and support will occur if frontline workers change the way they behave towards persons with dementia, their family members and supporters. This idea is a myth, a fallacy, and serves only to pin responsibility for poor practice unfairly on the practitioners. The more complicated truth of the matter is that practitioners work as members of a team, and so there is this area of team responsibility to consider.

In addition, practitioners work within settings, the design, staffing and resourcing of which are decided by other members of the organisation who do not work in these settings. They share responsibility, too, for the quality of dementia care and support that is provided. Beyond the 'local' teams, there are NHS trusts, and the national head offices of private companies and voluntary sector organisations. For many dementia care and support practitioners, there are also government departments and the government itself who share responsibility for the quality of dementia care and support which is provided to any one person with dementia, and their family members and supporters.

Let me be clear, this brief analysis of responsibility is not to minimise the crucial, central role and responsibility that dementia care and support practitioners have. Indeed, the focus of this book is on just how practitioners can achieve high-quality dementia care and support. Yet, the conditions in which frontline practitioners work, the working context, are not all within their gift. Neither is their pay, which in most cases tends to offer an instructive indication of the low value attributed to practitioners and the work they do with persons with dementia, family members and supporters.

The responsibility for the quality of dementia care and support lies at all levels of an organisation. It is everyone's responsibility. Yet, the problem with it being everyone's responsibility, without clear accountability, is that it becomes essentially no one's responsibility. This book is primarily about encouraging dementia care practitioners to view their crucial work in particular ways, via a critical relationship-centred approach, so that they can understand better how to take their responsibilities seriously. What is needed, in my view, is an equal focus on all of those whose decisions and actions impact on dementia care and support practice. In this I set a challenge to all organisations to take an organisational approach, to take organisational responsibility for the care and support which is provided in their name. This requires accountability for everyone and new approaches. In Chapter 8, an outline is given of a new approach to consider.

I look forward to seeing organisations respond to this. In the meantime, what follows are some suggestions about how care and support practitioners can push this agenda forwards by following a 'down-up' approach. This is an approach that is underpinned by care and support practitioners' practical experiences of dementia.

Placing any additional burden on dementia care and support practitioners' workloads is unfair and unrealistic. The clear sense I get from my conversations with practitioners is that they will do what they can to improve the quality of care and support they provide. I have often finished teaching or training sessions with an explicit recognition of this and acknowledgement of the perceived intangible barriers they face. Remember the image of practitioners shaking their heads and folding their arms from Chapter 4? The institutional barriers they identify are intangible ones, not least because some practitioners perceive there to be 'risk' associated with raising their concerns or sharing what they know with more senior members of the organisation by whom they are employed.

It comes out something like this: 'Do what you can do when you can do it.' The sentiment is as much an echo of what practitioners say more or less represents their own approach, as much as it is a reminder that persons with dementia, often voiceless in determining quality of care and support, will be the beneficiaries of their efforts. Now, 'Do what you can do when you can do it' isn't the most upbeat message that I could give to encourage practitioners to make positive change in dementia care and support. It is a pragmatic message and personally unsatisfactory when dementia care and support practitioners suggest what needs addressing is the status quo. However, pragmatism does not have to lack ambition about or action for radical change. The idea of the practitioner searching for opportunities to make a difference and then taking those opportunities is one that I have discussed with Alison Gordon, an experienced dementia care practitioner who has led and developed new services in dementia care and support over the past 25 years.

It is worth sharing Alison's thoughts about the kinds of qualities she feels practitioners need in order to work positively within, seemingly, ever resource-poor dementia care and support services. In conversation, Alison advanced the idea of the 'dementia passionista' and below is her description of this type of practitioner. It is followed by some more recent thoughts on the positive potential of dementia care and support practitioners provided by Natasha Wilson, Dementia Partnerships Officer for Age UK Sheffield.

> A passionista is more than a 'champion' or leader, it's not something you can learn or a skill you can gain from attending a workshop or course. Maybe it's something that may lie dormant within you and is triggered by a person, an event or a meeting of minds; maybe it's something that grows over a period of time. Maybe it's within us all and some people never trigger and release the enthusiasm that lies within.
>
> The features of a passionista are exuberance, passion, and an ability to motivate and influence others to change the way people with dementia are viewed and treated by the general public and others working within the care sector. A passionista creatively devises and shares a vision of excellence in dementia, stands firm in their beliefs and fights for the rights, perhaps sometimes triggering others' enthusiasm and creating ripples and waves that widen and spread out, often challenging the negativities in others and over time chipping away at installed negative beliefs. Can a passionista survive in this climate?

Natasha Wilson is also an experienced practitioner and a regular contributor to social media (@N_Wilson94 on Twitter), with her reportage on what it means to work passionately in offering care and support to persons with dementia. I asked Natasha to read Alison's definition of the 'dementia passionista' and then give her view on what she makes of this kind of dementia care and support practitioner. This is her view:

One that doesn't call themselves that would be where I would start. To me, it is somebody who has always inherently known this was their vocation/calling/life mission. Whatever you want to call it, you just know. It's always been there and there was no questioning that this is where you were going to be. I think that can be entirely coincidental/unexplainable, because of somebody special in your life, or because of somebody inspirational who sparks an awareness and consciousness in you that forces you to take action. Fortunately, I think all three apply to me personally.

From personal experience, the people who genuinely bring joy and meaning to people with dementia's lives have been people who truly know how to be human. Not compassionate, knowledgeable, empathetic, good communicators (obviously they embody all of these qualities, but in a way that is so subtle, genuine and natural that you know it is just the sum of who they are innately). They are the people with fantastic senses of humour, those who tell stories, those who light up a room, those who dare to really 'go there' with others. They laugh, they cry, they embrace, they dance, and they do so with all people. They categorically know that people living with dementia are just people – wonderful, funny, inspiring, deep, flawed, kind, struggling people, just like you and me. The only 'difference', if you can call it that, is the way in which all of the above, and more, manifest physically and emotionally, when certain chemicals and certain proteins behave in certain ways.

The people who belong to this 'tribe', as I will call it, hate red tape which causes emotional and professional distancing, which is so common and so harmful to anyone, including people living with dementia. They embed family values and behaviours in all aspects of life. And that, in reality, turns out to be the seemingly most basic actions, which in turn are unbelievably critical in ensuring people with dementia know they matter, are special, are unique and are loved.

I'd like to think I try my very hardest to be one of 'those people' in 'that tribe' on a daily basis in my role as 'dementia partnership officer and wellbeing centre lead'– far too waffly for my liking. Basically, I love my job more than anything and try to make other people less afraid to 'go there' with people, while hopefully making around 70 older people with dementia belly laugh and smile on a weekly basis. I think the little things I enjoy doing enrich my life and theirs equally. I love having families round to my house to share Sunday dinner with my own family; I like inviting families to my annual family BBQ; I like chatting on the phone to people on evenings/weekends (because surprisingly dementia doesn't quite operate on a 9–5 basis like a lot of services do). On the whole, I unashamedly love spending time with people who mean a great deal to me. They are my friends. Genuinely. It's just coincidental that some are 26, some are male, some are female, some live with dementia, some are my relatives, some are married, and so I could go on.

Why are we so afraid to forge genuine relationships with genuinely lovely people? I don't think that's such a radical or 'out there' concept?

Alison's notion of the 'dementia passionista' and Natasha's ideas of the 'tribe' are, in a sense, as one in describing a practitioner who realises they are likely to be working in adverse consequences, where the problems that arise do not, so far as is possible, deter the practitioner from the main focus of their work: *as a fellow human being*, understanding and meeting the needs of persons with dementia and their family members and supporters. The 'dementia passionista' is not simply a problem-solver but someone actively seeking to innovate, to find ways to get things done. It is a self-identification, requiring unambiguous awareness of the value in what you do. It is not a status that others can bestow on a practitioner but one that comes from within, directed by a kind of 'moral contract' between them and the person with dementia and their family members and supporters.

It is a moral contract because it is a choice a practitioner makes to be conscientiously attentive to excellence in care and support and to deliver on existing responsibilities to advocate on behalf of persons with dementia, their family members and supporters. The 'dementia passionista' will, if necessary, be the practitioner who asks the awkward questions, puts their head above the parapet to raise concerns or create new connections where these are beneficial and, in short, who uses the energy they have because of their passion for dementia care and support to 'do what you can do when you can do it'!

Natasha's ideas exist in the same space, part of the same 'tribe', and include valuing wholeheartedly and unashamedly the friendship, companionship and pure pleasure of being able to share. Is 'going there' another way of expressing something like a moral contract? I think it is. This message of doing what you can when you can, when viewed through the lens of Alison's 'dementia passionista' and Natasha's promise to 'go there', is reframed radically as a mutually life-affirming, progressive, activity. A focus, an identity, is created.

Some might argue here that I'm presenting an overly 'romanticised' vision for practitioners or that I'm seeking merely to rehash the hackneyed idea of 'carer as superhero'. There are certainly important reminders to be given about the importance of maintaining appropriate professional boundaries and about ensuring that you access what peer support and other forms of resources you might need to ensure you maintain your sense of wellbeing. These important reminders aside, I believe the 'dementia passionista' idea and the power in the commitment to 'go there' outweigh a lot of the possible objections, because of the need for dementia care and support practitioners to have a sense of identity that is specific to dementia care and support. Of course, this can come from role models within practice settings or organisations. In the absence of those people to inspire you, I give you Alison Gordon and Natasha Wilson.

Remember, much of the dementia care and support that is provided is not by nurses or social workers or doctors – those with established professional identities – but by support workers, domiciliary care workers, 'domestics', volunteers, those whose role providing dementia care and support is not necessarily easily discerned and acknowledged. The 'dementia passionista' is a role for anyone in dementia care and support to think about, to adopt. In short, anyone can decide to be a 'dementia passionista' or a member of the 'dementia tribe'.

One of the potential benefits of an orientation towards care and support which imagines a moral contract with persons with dementia, their family members and supporters is very straightforward. It is job satisfaction. It is to know, when you look at yourself in the mirror, that you did what you could, when you could do it. There is nothing in the idea of the 'dementia passionista' or 'dementia tribe' that suggests not doing your job as described in your contract of employment – it is essential that you do so. Rather, it is looking to reframe what you do towards action – action that offers benefits to persons with dementia, their family members and supporters. Starting with the example that you set, an enhanced notion of personal leadership begins to unfold, beyond the responsibilities you have to be lead participant in communication-based care and support relationships.

It is to possible directions for developing this enhanced personal leadership role that I now turn, and the other relationships practitioners have within and, potentially outside, their particular dementia care or support setting. Remember, 'enhanced personal leadership' is something that everyone can demonstrate. This is because there are no absolutes, no magnitude of leadership that is too big or too small. Any personal leadership has the potential to bring about positive change. The challenge is the same for everyone and the reward is likely to be personal, too: do what you can do when you can do it!

One dimension of the practical experience of dementia care and support is that of practitioners working with colleagues in their respective settings. Following the arguments made so far, each practitioner must consider themselves to be a member of their dementia care and support practitioner community. By extension, if not already the case, practitioners must view their colleagues as being engaged in the same or related care and support activity that they are. Using the relationship-centred approach outlined in this book, colleagues are each in the same position as you, having 'lead participant' status in their interactions with persons with dementia, family members or supporters. However, it is important to note that this approach does not rely on only one practitioner dealing with a specific person, their family member or supporter. It does depend on the setting and the nature of care and support, but it is likely, if not inevitable, that a number of practitioners within a dementia practitioner community will interact with any one person with dementia, family member or supporter.

Some settings and organisations will operate a 'named nurse' or 'key worker' system to promote continuity of care and support and allocation of 'workload' to staff members. Even if this is the case, shift-systems, rota requirements, annual leave and sickness absence will mean that practitioners share responsibility for any one person's care and support. Overall, the result is that within the community of dementia care and support practice there will be a need to share information between themselves about a person with dementia and their family members or supporters.

This is where protocols, such as 'This is me' (Alzheimer's Society, 2020d), can be seen to offer great benefits. A quick way of comprehending key biographical, preference and family and support network information – so long as this has been completed accurately and is accessible to practitioners who might need it – can be tremendously valuable. Therefore, one thing that can be done is to check, if this has not already been done, whether or not the 'This is me' form is being used and, if so, whether or not everyone within your community of practice knows where to find it, how to complete it and then actually uses it.

As was also noted in Chapter 3, the suggestion to imagine 'walking in the footsteps' of family members and supporters invites questions about what their needs might be. For example, awareness of John's Campaign (2020) was argued to offer family members and supporters greater access to their loved ones in hospitals and information on how their needs are met within the setting. A further action, and, therefore, a further example of enhanced personal leadership, would be to initiate a discussion with fellow practitioners about the kind of support and guidance you offer family members and supporters. This collective discussion and sharing of perspectives might lead to improvements in the support and guidance made available but, remember, it does not have to be the lone practitioner who takes responsibility for doing this. Raising the issue might be the extent of your contribution on this matter, so long as a potential improvement like this is considered or acted on by somebody. However, it might well be you who is asked to do this. Do so only if you feel you can and, if so, consider first who might be able to help you do it most effectively from either inside or outside your own practice community.

On the issue of more than one practitioner interacting with a person with dementia, each is likely to learn things which the other would find equally useful. Each organisation will have its own paperwork and administrative practices, and these might already provide a solution to this issue. However, it may not, and a question then arises about how what is learned from a person with dementia, or, indeed, from a family member or supporter, is shared. From my own research, it was suggested that care practitioners may retain rather than share knowledge they gain through their interactions with persons with dementia and their family members or supporters. Retained as 'working knowledge', rather than shared systematically in writing or verbally to colleagues as a whole, this represents insights which, when viewing the practitioner community, could be considered 'information leaks'.

The practitioner, recognising their links and responsibilities to sustain the collective knowledge of their community of dementia care and support practitioners, might decide to explore with those colleagues how such information and knowledge is recorded and how it might be useful to find ways, if none exist currently, to maximise its capture and use by everyone in that community of practice. Clearly, if the information has been shared by a person with a practitioner on a confidential basis, then careful judgement is required about the appropriateness of sharing this with others. How this is decided is another question but, again, could be raised with colleagues within the practice community for a collective best-practice decision and consistent approach.

As you will have ideas about how to improve care and support so, it should be assumed, do your colleagues. One of the most powerful results of viewing yourself as part of a community of practitioners is to see how knowledge, expertise, insights and passion for driving change are multiplied. By valuing your own expertise and that of your colleagues, it is possible to begin to see new potential in working collaboratively to improve dementia care and support.

But yours is only one community of dementia care and support practitioners to which you belong. There are others. Depending on your organisation, there are likely to be similar communities operating locally, regionally or nationally. In similar ways to those suggested for your own team or community of practice, these other communities offer a resource for you to access and learn from – but with the insights provided by a different, unique combination of practitioners. So, a further example of an enhanced leadership role might be to seek to make contact with other communities of practitioners within your own organisation and then you, or a better placed colleague, might explore the ways you might pool your expertise, resources or ideas to draw fresh approaches and impetus into your practice area. In short, practitioners must seek to learn from each other.

For example, I was involved in facilitating a Dementia Champions conference in 2015 in South Yorkshire. It was part of the South Yorkshire Dementia Creative Arts Exhibition (2020) that year. The conference was a new attempt to bring together dementia care and support practitioners who were working in NHS trusts to encourage sharing of innovation and expertise among different communities of practice. Just to note, not all participants in this conference were formally designated as 'dementia champions' but all had taken or held some form of lead responsibility for dementia care and support. Could you help initiate new forms of sharing between your known practitioner communities at conference-like events?

Such acts are simply an extension of the recognition that others working as practitioners have insights, knowledge, ideas and ambitions that are worth knowing for your own practice. In a sense, it requires you to expand your view of which dementia communities you actually belong to. Then, the challenge is to find ways of creating opportunities to learn from each other and support each other. In seeking to forge and maintain these links, identifying effective ways of communicating with each other, there is also the possibility of developing aspects of dementia care practice and support across a range of connected services. Where once you may have felt isolated, there arises the possibility of creating new understanding and collective approaches which originate in and grow as a result of the expertise and action of dementia care and support practitioners. The significance of being part of a wider community of learning and of practice should now be fairly clear.

There is, in this 'down-up' approach, the possibility of joining with others to discuss and debate what is needed to improve care and support offered to persons with dementia and their families and supporters. Within any organisation, it will be harder to ignore proposals for change that numerous practitioners – as opposed to individual practitioners – have identified and come to agreement about. As I have noted previously, there may exist mechanisms within your organisation which serve the same purpose and are considered to be effective. However, if they do not exist or seem ineffective, then taking on this type of enhanced personal leadership role will promote opportunities for practitioners to share their expertise and the intelligence they collectively possess. The tantalising prospect is of helping to improve the care and support offered to persons with dementia and their family members and supporters.

Such action will make it more likely than not that those with formal leadership responsibilities within organisations will have credible ways of knowing where problems and/or solutions lie for the provision of dementia care and support. Offering strategic or clinical managers this resource – and avoiding the temptation to dwell on why they had not sought to know this themselves if they have not – advances the likelihood that persons with dementia and their family members and supporters will see positive change. Of course, this kind of initiative, like the others previously suggested, offers no guarantee of success. But, you would have done what you could do when you could do it. Others, as suggested in the call for organisations to take greater responsibility for the quality of care and support provided in their name, may need their own kinds of encouragement to begin to view themselves more as part of the wider dementia care and support community.

The final extension of the notion of practice community that I would like you to consider is, again, inspired by the invitation to 'walk in our footsteps' which came from those affected by dementia. As should be clear, 'dementia' refers to a diverse collection of individuals, and ranges from those with little or no cognitive impairment, who are more or less independent, to those whose impairments are so severe that they are heavily, if not totally, reliant on care and support. One of the repeated findings of research which seeks to understand better 'the dementia pathway' (i.e. how persons with dementia and their significant others move between services and sources of support) is that it is too often fractured, poorly coordinated and not at all really what a pathway is generally agreed to mean (Care Quality Commission, 2014; Alzheimer's Society, 2016).

In England, the situation was unlikely to have been helped by the hiatus following what could well go down in history as its first and last national dementia strategy (Department of Health, 2009). This five-year strategy document, with 17 recommendations, was a tremendous catalyst for service improvement but, curiously, did not include within it a commitment to evaluate its own outcomes. A shift to a local/regional focus for dementia strategy has since occurred via a number of stepping stones (e.g. NHS England, 2014; Department of Health, 2015). In contrast, Scotland is approaching the end of its third National Dementia Strategy (Scottish Government, 2017) and Wales is in the middle of a four-year Dementia Action Plan (Welsh Government, 2018). In Northern Ireland, a regional strategy for improving dementia services (Health, Social Services and Public Safety, 2011) is the most recent document of its kind on the Department of Health website.

In England, NHS clinical commissioning groups, NHS trusts

and local authorities, along with key partners from the voluntary sector and others (e.g. National Dementia Action Alliance, 2020), have developed multi-agency dementia strategy groups and local dementia strategies (e.g. NHS Sheffield Clinical Commissioning Group, 2019; Southern Health NHS Foundation Trust, 2019). This kind of approach provides an informed means by which to commission geographically specific services which offer identifiable routes for people affected by dementia to access timely information and advice, peer group support, as well as a range of activities to encourage good physical and mental health for all affected by dementia.

These dementia strategy groups have a very important potential role to play in building and articulating meaningful pathways for those affected by dementia in specific localities. As a practitioner, what can you learn from all of this? I argue that as a dementia care practitioner you are also a member of this wider community of service providers, outside your organisation, operating in the area where you work. These other service providers contain other practitioners, just like you, who have the same goals in mind. They have expertise, knowledge, skills and resources which are likely to be of great value to you and to the other members of your practice community. Therefore, having a reasonable understanding of your local dementia community of providers, your local dementia strategy and any coherent pathway it has suggested will allow you to share this with colleagues and with persons with dementia, their family members and supporters. There is likely, for example, to be information and advice available on websites or in paper form, which these organisations would be only too willing for you to access in order that persons with dementia, their family members and supporters can be well informed, and thereby empowered, by knowing what options are available to them.

All that is required is a quick internet search or a phone call in order to plug yourself and your practice community into the wider local dementia community and the significant resources they hold. This, like all the suggested actions of an enhanced leadership role, only requires your motivation and a little time. It may be that someone else with more time could do it, if you suggest it. Beginning to engage proactively like this is easier if you perceive yourself to be a 'dementia passionista' or someone who is willing to 'go there' and, also, by realising that you are a significant member of the wider dementia community of practice, as well as your own organisation's practice communities and your own practice community where you work.

Summary

In this chapter, the practical experience of the dementia care or support practitioner has been elaborated. Care has been taken to apportion overall responsibility for dementia care and support outcomes to organisations, and not to individual practitioners. An invitation was made for organisational approaches which take the sharing out of responsibility seriously. Dementia care and support practitioners were invited to imagine their roles through the lens of Alison Gordon's notion of the 'dementia passionista' and Natasha Wilson's vision of the 'dementia tribe'. This orientation towards actively pursuing positive change was described as a form of moral contract with persons with dementia, their family members and supporters. Forms of enhanced leadership action were invited, too, and this was suggested to be easier if practitioners acknowledged their membership of three types of related dementia practice communities. These are their immediate practice community, located in their work setting; their organisation's practice community – other singular practice communities within the same organisation; and the local practice community, comprised of multi-agency organisations with a common aim of supporting persons with dementia, their family members and supporters.

In the next chapter, the focus turns to yet further practice communities. They are those which determine quality standards in dementia care and support and those which make recommendations about dementia education and training. With it being argued throughout this book so far that 'expertise' resides with those most affected by dementia, and 'learning' is what goes on between these experts, how does this compare with expert knowledge and learning as defined by 'policy'?

CHAPTER 7

Engaging with Dementia Standards Communities

In this chapter, the focus shifts towards a discussion of quality and standards in dementia care and support and recommendations about dementia education. Questions are asked about where the expertise of dementia care and support practitioners, and, to a lesser extent, that of persons with dementia and family carers and supporters, is recognised in these important domains of influence and knowledge. Key limitations in current approaches are suggested, alongside proposals for how these might be addressed.

As the end of the book approaches, it is perhaps useful to reiterate that the intention behind it is to contribute to ideas about how to approach dementia care and support. It's quite a crowded space already and, as I stated at the outset, I do not believe there is a single approach which asks or seeks to answer all of the questions practitioners have about services and support for persons with dementia, their family members and supporters. How could there be when there is so much diversity among persons with dementia and family members and their supporters? How could there be with such a range of places and settings in which care and support is offered? How could there be when 'practitioners' represents such a diverse group of professionals, each with their private and practical experiences of dementia which might influence what they do?

As a critical consumer of dementia knowledge, you already know all of this. There will be some ideas which, intuitively, make sense. There will be others that seem remote and 'too theoretical'. Where you locate the ideas about a critical, relationship-centred approach to dementia care and support is for you to decide. In writing about what I have learned, I have attempted to explain things as clearly as I can. I am not presenting a 'theory' that I want practitioners to feel they should 'adopt', like some mantra that interferes with your normal critical faculties. I invite you to consider the arguments that I've made. At most, if they chime with your own understandings and offer new possibilities for you to enhance the care and support you provide to persons with dementia and their families and supporters, then that would be a 'win' as far as I am concerned. Other ideas and approaches are available.

There is, however, a little more I would like you to consider by way of extending the critical, relationship-centred approach. The focus on the practical domain of experience in the previous chapter took discussion into the notion of 'practice communities', the groups of practitioners to which you belong. Making links with these communities of dementia practice has the potential to bring many benefits to you and your own practice – and vice versa. Yet, there are other 'communities' to which you belong which are less tangible but nonetheless important. These dementia communities are the practice standards and guidance communities and the dementia education and training communities.

This may seem like a long-winded way of explaining things but it is deliberately so. I believe that as a dementia care and support practitioner, you have a responsibility to acknowledge your membership of the key groups that issue dementia care and support standards and guidance and those groups which issue recommendations about dementia education and training. The long-windedness is necessary because I suspect many dementia care and support practitioners view these 'standard setting' groups and their work as remote and nothing to do with them. By this, I am certainly not suggesting that practitioners do not follow standards and best practice guidelines or are not interested in attending training or accessing educational opportunities.

I do, however, suggest that you may think that you have no contribution to make to the work these groups do or have no right to contribute. You would be wrong on both counts. While more is said later about your potential contribution, it is worth being aware that when guidance and standards are being written or reviewed an invitation is made for contributions from anyone who considers themselves to be a 'stakeholder'. If you believe that the work of these groups is nothing to do with you, it might be because you have not seen the 'guidance in consultation' list that is updated on the respective websites of key organisations, such as the one for the National Institute for Health and Care Excellence (2020b).

It is the same for everyone: if you want to make a difference, you have to get involved. These websites of statutory organisations give options for you to sign up to email alerts which flag new guidance or standards that are in consultation or published, along with other ways to participate (e.g. National Institute for Health and Care Excellence, 2020c, 2020d). I am not a dementia care or support practitioner but I am very interested in guidance and standards. I imagine you are, too. One of the ways that dementia care and support practitioners can value their own expertise is by sharing it within guidance and standards communities.

Dementia care and support standards

These are the guidance and quality standards that it is recommended should inform the nature, quality and delivery of dementia care and support where you work. Are you personally aware of the guidance and quality standards that apply to your dementia care and support setting? If you are, that's great. Does everyone in your practice setting know about them as well? If you don't know the guidance and quality standards, though it might be someone else's responsibility to have made you aware, what are you going to do about it?

There are clear advantages to knowing which guidelines and standards apply to your care or support setting and what they stipulate. These dementia guidelines (e.g. National Institute for Health and Care Excellence, 2015, 2018) and quality standards (e.g. National Institute for Health and Care Excellence, 2019) contain important, evidence-based, recommendations about what you and your team should be seeking to achieve. There are wide-ranging recommendations, and so it should be possible to find some which apply to your specific role and service. All dementia care and support services are expected to take these national recommendations into account in the design and delivery of services. Knowing them will benefit you and your practice community and increase the likelihood that persons with dementia, their family members and supporters have their rightful expectations met for quality of care and support.

A second advantage, which is alluded to above, is that guidance and quality standards offer a 'neutral' but authoritative form of leverage. For example, if you and your colleagues feel that no one is listening to your concerns or suggestions for improvement and these concerns or suggestions are supported by recommendations made in guidance and quality standards, then a route is provided to add credence to your practice communities' perspectives and voice. Wider awareness that services do not follow or meet national recommendations is generally undesirable for organisations. It is, arguably, a dementia care practitioner's responsibility to raise this with those in their respective organisations, be it indirectly via a practice manager or directly if that option is unavailable or is judged, after sharing, to have been ineffective.

Remember, the idea of the 'dementia passionista' outlined in Chapter 6 includes advocating on behalf of persons with dementia, their family members and supporters. Equally, it is to seek to do this through collaboration and not with combativeness. Imagining how your contribution is likely to be received should guide you in deciding how to do this. Even better, a discussion within your practice setting to build a consensus about raising any matters would be a sensible course of action to take.

So far, it has been argued that dementia care practitioners should view themselves as members of dementia care and support guidance and standards communities, and it has been suggested that you find and engage with these groups, to share your expertise and help shape the important documents these statutory organisations produce. It has also been noted that the work you do in your practice setting should reflect the appropriate guidance and standards. If you are unaware of what this guidance is, it is recommended that you find out. Knowledge of guidance and standards can support you as practitioners to make more robust cases for change. For example: 'We need more time and resources in our practice area because that would help us to meet the recommended standards for dementia care, which state that...'

The triadic model of relationship-centred dementia care and support suggests there are at least three domains where you can seek further knowledge in order to meet the needs of persons with dementia, their family members and supporters. In the points made above, which refer to the domain of the practitioner, the notion of practical experience is expanded to include knowledge of, participation in and benchmarking using the outputs of dementia guidance and standards communities.

Guidance, standards and advice is also produced by organisations of persons with dementia (e.g. Dementia Alliance

International, 2016; Dementia Engagement and Empowerment Project, 2020c) and by organisations representing family members and supporters (e.g. Age UK, 2020a; Carers Trust, 2020; Caring for the Carers, 2020). By recognising these other kinds of communities which are both credible and produce guidance and standards, there are further discussions which might be had within your practice community, if they are made available. The main difference, it should be remembered, is that statutory guidance and recommendations on standards *must* be considered. Therefore, other forms of guidance from groups representing persons with dementia and carers and supporters have potentially less traction. It is worth also remembering then that these alternatives, authored by experts in their experiences of dementia, will have zero traction if dementia care and support practitioners do not know about them, access them and read and share them in order to consider their value.

Dementia education and training standards

Attention now turns to dementia education and training. The direction I now take might not seem, at first glance, to be directly relevant to some of the ideas covered up to this point. However, education and training is clearly very important in dementia care and support practice. Yet, I appreciate it might feel a little unusual being drawn into thinking about your role in the recommendations that exist for dementia education and training. Maybe this will help. In the section above, the focus is on *your* guidance and standards. These are concerned with statutory recommendations about *what* dementia and care and support should be provided and *how* it should be delivered in practice. In shifting focus towards dementia education and training, it is a move to think about and discuss what education and training providers are recommended to teach. Put another way, these are recommendations about *what you need to know about dementia* to be a dementia care and support practitioner.

There is a vast range of dementia education and training providers, including, in no particular order, universities, training companies, voluntary sector organisations and in-house training departments located within organisations. A starting point for opening up education and training for discussion is to follow up on the principle outlined in this book – that is, in my view, persons with dementia, family members and supporters and dementia care and support practitioners are the experts in their experiences of dementia. So, my question is: where is this expertise acknowledged and drawn upon in the recommendations about what dementia knowledge educators and trainers should teach?

Answers to this question lie in looking carefully at *what* this guidance states but, also, at *who* has provided the expertise for the formulation of the education and training recommendations. I should admit at this point that I have an unease about being told what to do, what to teach and how to teach it. I have a critical view of most things, looking for the cons, as well as the pros. But, as someone with some teaching experience, I feel an inclination to discover what is required within a particular episode of education or training, by interacting with those present. Seeking to understand what is needed, rather than repeating what has been decided elsewhere, should be learned. Prescriptive approaches make teaching fairly redundant. So in that regard I have an axe to grind, but it is one specific to dementia because of what I have previously argued: that 'dementia' claims and claims about 'people with dementia' are hugely problematic. That is, unless you are happy to ignore this complexity.

Some historical context to the issue of dementia education and training is useful in understanding where we are now and how we have got here. In particular, this historical account permits examination of what dementia education and training is intended to achieve and, also, who has contributed to the expertise which now guides what dementia care and support practitioners are expected to know.

Historical account of dementia education and training in the UK

In terms of an interest in dementia education in the UK, the first serious report on the subject was published by the All-Party Parliamentary Group on Dementia (2009). This made seven recommendations, and among these, five called for enhancements to dementia education for health care providers:

- Prioritising objective 13 of the National Dementia Strategy for England, namely, an informed and effective workforce for people with dementia

- Shift to a situation where the workforce as a whole demonstrates effective knowledge and skills in caring for people with dementia

- Careful design of workforce development programmes so that the needs of care staff are met and the lives of people with dementia are improved

- Regulation of dementia care trainers to combat current inequalities in quality

- Greater recognition of the level of skill required to provide good quality dementia care as well as the importance of maximising the quality of life of individuals who develop dementia.

(All-Party Parliamentary Group on Dementia, 2009, p.xiv)

Shortly afterwards, the National Dementia Strategy (NDS) for

England (Department of Health, 2009) was published, and this stated a need to develop a 'skilled and effective' workforce (pp.65–67) in the form of a specific objective (Reid, 2009a). The main reasons given for this were that people with dementia and carers consulted as part of the NDS noted that care professionals often did not know how to diagnose effectively and also did not know 'what works' for people with dementia. A further reason presented was that given the majority of people with dementia lived in the community, it was vital that awareness of dementia and information which might be helpful was in place (Department of Health, 2009, p.44). The ambition of objective 13, to be delivered by joint commissioning between health and social care, was summed up as follows:

> People with dementia and their carers need to be supported and cared for by a trained workforce, with the right knowledge, skills and understanding of dementia to offer the best quality care and support. (Department of Health, 2009, p.66)

Tucked away in this section of the NDS were two suggestions for delivering this ambition for improvement to dementia care education. The first was the possibility of developing 'core competencies' (p.66) which care professionals would have to achieve, and the second was the development of some form of 'kite-marking' (p.67) of good practice in education to help health and care education commissioners determine their choice of providers. Both of these suggestions have since been taken up and expanded.

The first example was a document published by a government body outlining eight core competencies for social and health care professionals (Skills for Care & Skills for Health, 2011). This document makes a first attempt in the UK to name the areas of knowledge which it was felt social and health care professionals must possess in order to work effectively with people with dementia. These competencies are presented as 'principles', and the document suggests health care providers seek to embed them within their practice and training.

The principles are listed below:

Principle 1: Know the early signs of dementia.

Principle 2: Early diagnosis of dementia helps people receive information, support and treatment at the earliest possible stage.

Principle 3: Communicate sensitively to support meaningful interaction.

Principle 4: Promote independence and encourage activity.

Principle 5: Recognise the signs of distress resulting from confusion and respond by diffusing a person's anxiety and supporting their understanding of the events they experience.

Principle 6: Family members and other carers are valued, respected and supported just like those they care for and are helped to gain access to dementia care advice.

Principle 7: Managers need to take responsibility to ensure members of their team are trained and well supported to meet the needs of people with dementia.

Principle 8: Work as part of a multi-agency team to support the person with dementia.

(Skills for Care & Skills for Health, 2011, p.2)

The next concrete move towards developing a definitive curriculum for dementia education came from a group of academics who were members of the Higher Education for Dementia Network (HEDN). In 2013, HEDN published a Curriculum for UK Dementia Education (CfDE) (Higher Education for Dementia Network,

2013; see also Tsaroucha, Benbow, Kingston *et al.*, 2011). This was the first national guidance which gave recommendations about dementia content and learning outcomes for higher education programmes for health and social care staff. It was the outcome of a number of years' work by specific members of HEDN.

For example, Pulsford, Hope and Thompson (2007) undertook research to develop ideas for the development of a curriculum document. In a study of social work, adult and learning disability nursing programmes in the UK, they discovered that students received a mean of three hours' teaching related to dementia during their entire pre-registration programme.

While only 13 higher education institutions took part (of 26 reporting the provision of dementia education), the authors reported that 'taken as a whole, most courses are congruent with the recommendations of HEDN's dementia curriculum' (Pulsford, Hope and Thompson, 2007, p.11, and see Table 5 on page 9 for a list of early topics).

The CfDE (Higher Education for Dementia Network, 2013) was one of the underpinning sources for the Dementia Core Skills Education and Training Framework (Skills for Health, Skills for Care and Health Education England, 2015, updated 2018) which emerged shortly afterwards. This is presented as a 'comprehensive resource' and is a far more substantial document than the previous attempts to specify substantive areas of learning in dementia in England.

This document identifies not only areas of knowledge, and depth of knowledge, but matches these to so-called 'workforce groups'. These groups are Tier 1, 'awareness', 'relevant to the entire health and care workforce'; Tier 2, 'fundamental', 'relevant to all health and health and care staff in settings where they are likely to have regular contact with people affected by dementia'; and Tier 3, 'leadership', 'relevant to staff working intensively with people affected by dementia including those who take a lead in decision making' (Skills for Health, Skills for Care and Health Education England, 2015, p.11). It is worth highlighting the stated intentions behind the document as a whole, which are to:

- standardise the interpretation of dementia education and training

- guide the focus and aims of dementia education and training delivery through key learning outcomes

- ensure the educational relevance of dementia training

- improve the quality and consistency of education and training provision.

(Skills for Health, Skills for Care and Health Education England, 2015, p.9)

The momentum towards 'standardisation' continued with a Health Education England initiative, 'What works in dementia training and education?' (Surr and Gates, 2016; Surr, Gates, Irving *et al.*, 2016). This further extension represents, fundamentally, a process whereby certain topics of dementia knowledge are valued above others and, in the final analysis, 'prescribed'. 'What works in dementia training and education?' was a three-phase project. The first phase was to survey all higher education institutions to discover what dementia education provision exists. The second phase was to contact the survey respondents and encourage them to map their individual dementia education modules against the multiple learning outcomes for all 14 'subjects' of the Dementia Core Skills Education and Training Framework (Skills for Health, Skills for Care and Health Education England, 2015). The objective here was to identify the degree of congruence of existing provision with the 'subjects' posited within the Framework. The final phase of this project was for the research team to conduct a small number of higher education institution case studies in which the views and perspectives of all key stakeholders were sought (Surr and Gates, 2016).

As someone who was asked to undertake the phase 2 task, I can report that I received the lengthy draft text for each 'subject' and was, indeed, encouraged to locate elements of the course I ran at the time within this wide-ranging framework. Alarm bells rang. The realisation crystallised that a 'script' for authorised dementia education was close to being finalised. I knew that there was an ambition to develop a 'kite-marking' approach within the commissioning of dementia education (Department of Health, 2009), and so it struck me that within a short space of time it would not be viable for higher education institutions to develop dementia education courses which did not align with required topics contained within the Framework.

I had two objections. The first was that higher education institutions are, traditionally, places where academic freedom is protected. A 'national curriculum' for dementia delivered in higher education institutions must mean that this freedom (e.g. to innovate, to develop course content with local stakeholders – including dementia care and support practitioners – and to disagree with the 'national curriculum') is sacrificed, or else the 'business' is lost to another education or training provider. The Framework does not specify *how* topics should be taught but, in specifying *what*, it seemed to me that dementia training, rather than dementia education, had become the height of ambition presumed for dementia care and support practitioners (Reid, 2009b), a position that appeared to be endorsed by the Higher Education for Dementia Network (Surr, Baillie, Waugh *et al.*, 2016).

My second objection, relating to the preceding point, was that it was noted that one of the stated intentions of the Dementia Core Skills Education and Training Framework was to 'ensure the educational relevance of dementia training'. The discussions with a small number of practitioners reported earlier (Chapter 4) suggest that what is needed to improve dementia care is not 'deliverable' by frontline dementia care and support practitioners alone. For me, it raises the prospect that a false and simplistic assumption underpins the Framework initiative – that providing dementia care and support practitioners with 'national curriculum in dementia' training will deliver better outcomes for persons with dementia, their families and supporters. For the reasons noted above, I have to disagree.

Who decides what is learned?

Discussions about dementia curricula do make mention of people affected by dementia being consulted as part of the discussions (e.g. Pulsford, Hope and Thompson, 2007; Department of Health, 2009; Skills for Health, Skills for Care and Health Education England, 2015). However, it is not clear that any research has been undertaken to seek to understand what persons with dementia and their family members or supporters feel that health and social care professionals need to know about dementia (e.g. Reid and Witherspoon, 2008) or, indeed, what frontline dementia care and support practitioners feel they need to know.

The notion that persons with dementia, family members and dementia care and support practitioners might have something to contribute to these discussions about dementia education seems uncontroversial. Yet, while academic research in dementia over the past 25 years has increasingly involved those affected in order to learn from their experiences, there has been little evidence of a similar appetite for inclusion of key stakeholders in the development of dementia education standards. There are many examples of where persons with dementia have been involved in undertaking educational consultation or have been directly involved in training (e.g. EDUCATE, 2020; Sheffield

Dementia Involvement Group, 2020). However, there appears to be a gap here, and it would be in keeping with Post's (2001) notion of developing an 'epistemology of humility' to seek to examine whether what is being suggested about dementia education by government bodies and dementia educators is what persons with dementia, family members and supporters and care and support practitioners actually prioritise. Is the debate about a national dementia curriculum going on without those who the most significant expertise?

Summary

Dementia care and support practitioners are expected to apply national recommendations, guidance and quality standards. It is unclear whether these were informed by dementia care and support practitioners. They are also subject to recommendations about what they should know about dementia to do their jobs. Yet, dementia care and support practitioners were not, it seems, consulted about their needs, nor was their expertise sought in formulating these recommendations. What does this suggest about the value of dementia care and support practitioners, and about whose 'expertise' is most influential in standard-setting for services and for education and training?

It must be that those who are considered the 'experts' are experts only because they have learned from persons with dementia, from family members and supporters and from dementia care and support practitioners. There is, it seems, a crisis of representation for dementia care and support practitioners in the formulation of dementia policy. Why is this? Might it be that practitioners would say 'we can't do that' or 'we don't need to know that'? How might this expertise upset things? Well, some 'experts' might lose their position of influence, a change to the status quo. The views might expose a praxis gap, a challenge to the notion that anything's possible in dementia care and support if practitioners receive training. This might mean that the policy aspirations might be made to look a little unrealistic. A policy with reduced but realistic ambitions might be required. The education 'experts' might also find themselves with less representation and power, necessitating a further realignment of how things are normally done.

Yet, I have started to believe that there is another route which might be more fruitful. I think that it is already under construction. Appropriately, perhaps, I was prompted to think about this by one of the most obvious omissions I could see in the Dementia Core Skills Education and Training Framework – that is, no suggestions are made about how the education and training topics can be most effectively taught. The focus instead is on the 'what'. For me, *how* dementia education and training is taught is of huge concern. In the book so far, I have made it clear what my views are about this. Practitioners learn from persons with dementia and from family members and supporters. They also learn by reflecting on their practice and from the practice communities of which they are a member. By starting here, it is clear who has the expertise and it is also clear who is doing the real teaching.

I have come to the conclusion that persons with dementia, family members and supporters should be encouraged, supported and paid to teach practitioners about dementia. This sort of formalising of the teacher role already occurs in some education and training, though whether payment commensurate with lecturer or expert speaker status occurs is a question for elsewhere. I believe payment should be at this level. I have encouraged and supported persons with dementia and family members to teach, face-to-face, on education courses I have run. I have consulted persons with dementia, family members and care practitioners about what to include on education courses. But the idea that has germinated for me goes beyond the idea of partial or sporadic involvement of the dementia experts in the design and delivery of education and training. It involves the dementia experts claiming their expertise from universities, training companies, voluntary sector organisations and in-house training companies. My idea of a different way for doing dementia education and training is for organisations to create their own 'University of Dementia', owned, run and led by those most affected by dementia.

In the final chapter, this idea is expanded and is argued to be a logical extension of a critical, relationship-centred approach to dementia care and support, including, of course, dementia care and support practitioners.

education and training. It involves the dementia experts training their expertise more intensively, including companies, voluntary sector organisations and in-house training companies. My idea of a different way for existing dementia education and training is for organisations to create their own 'University of Dementia', owned, run and led by those most affected by dementia.

In the final chapter, this idea is expanded and is argued to be a logical extension of a critical, relationship-centred approach to dementia care and support, including, of course, dementia care and support practitioners.

CHAPTER 8

Doing Critical, Relationship-Centred Dementia Care and Support

The intention throughout this book has been to offer ideas about *doing* dementia care and support. It is in this active, practical sense of dementia care and support, *where* and *how* it occurs, that key relationships are made visible, offering themselves up for scrutiny and thought. In this way, the dementia care or support practitioner is identified as occupying the pivotal role in influencing the quality of care and support that is available to persons with dementia and their family members and supporters. In the preceding chapters, dementia care and support practitioners are invited to consider their role through the ideas associated with a critical, relationship-centred approach to dementia care and support. In particular, care and support practitioners have been encouraged to position persons with dementia, their family members and supporters – as well as themselves – as experts, possessing valuable knowledge. The logical extension of this view is to see dementia care as a process of learning and teaching – an educational cycle.

However, just because practitioners occupy this pivotal role does not mean that they should or can have exclusive responsibility for the overall quality of dementia services and support. Though practitioners may sometimes feel that they are 'to blame' for poor dementia care, the arguments made earlier (Chapters 6 and 7) make it clear that practitioners are members of communities of practice, and of organisations. In their normal roles, dementia care and support practitioners typically do not have direct influence over decisions made about staffing levels or the material resources available to them, such as the range of activities on offer in the setting or the built environment in which they work. Therefore, attempts to improve dementia care and support by individual practitioners are going to be limited in scope unless there are meaningful and transparent ways in which decision-makers listen to and act on the intelligence which frontline practitioners possess about how care and support can be improved. Individual practitioners can, do and should seek to make a difference. However, fundamental and sustainable positive change for all persons with dementia, their family members and supporters comes from within organisations, where responsibility ultimately resides.

If decision-makers within organisations really want to provide excellent dementia care and support, they have to engage and not wait to be engaged by those with the expertise to help them to achieve this. There are several changes that are required as a first step to this becoming a sustainable reality, where such practices are not already the norm. Most importantly, organisations have to wake up to the expertise of their dementia care and support practitioners, and their foundational role in the key 'business' of the organisation. It is also necessary to fully recognise the expertise of persons with dementia and their family members and supporters. Their collective expertise, their experiences of lives lived with dementia, is what is missing. This engagement is not synonymous with tokenistic rounds of service user consultation, attempting to give a serious impression of listening, but not really committed to acting on what is heard.

I believe that valuing and then engaging with the respective expertise of dementia care and support practitioners, and the persons with dementia they work with, and the family members or supporters of persons with dementia they also work with, is the most obvious route by which organisations might get close to former Prime Minister David Cameron's ambition for the UK to become 'the best place in the world to live with dementia'. This is, after all, what people in the UK feel they deserve. If you are a decision-maker, a senior manager, and want to make this vision a reality for your dementia care and support organisation, I suggest you plan your strategy with those who have the most credible expertise.

It is presumed throughout this book, perhaps unfairly, that dementia care and support organisations do not operate on this basis. Yet this simple approach to generating readily available intelligence to improve dementia care and support is at the core of the critical, relationship-centred approach which has been outlined in these pages. It is here, in this simple way of visualising how dementia care and support is actually done, that all organisations can create their own 'University of Dementia'. Everything that you need is in the knowledge possessed by those experts already within an organisation's orbit, or within the communities within which these experts have membership. Persons with dementia, family members and supporters and dementia care and support practitioners are all knowledgeable experts and can teach others what they know, if organisations are willing to listen, learn and act. There may or may not be value in bringing in education or training experts to facilitate or contribute to your university's work. That is a decision your 'University of Dementia' has to make, together.

Perhaps bringing in the traditional education and training 'experts' is not necessary. Why can't persons with dementia teach care and support practitioners about their care and support needs? Why can't family members and supporters teach practitioners about their needs and knowledge? Why can't dementia care and support practitioners teach directors or strategic managers about what does and does not work, and where opportunities for improvement exist? To me, it is incongruous that academic research studies consistently identify and outline the expertise these 'groups' possess, yet this expertise is rarely utilised within organisations whose business it is to do dementia care and support.

The focus of this book is the 'practitioner as expert' and their role in influencing the quality of dementia care and support. The starting point for encouraging practitioners to think more about this pivotal role, in what I describe as a 'down-up' approach to promoting positive change, and become more aware of how what they do makes a tremendous difference, is to encourage them to be critical in their consumption of dementia knowledge. The examples of the terms 'people with dementia' and 'dementia' were given to try and illustrate how easy it can be to slip into generalisations and lose the complexity when thinking and learning about persons with dementia and, consequently, family members and supporters, too. The term 'carers' was another example provided of a way in which the diversity of human beings is sacrificed for convenience, the cost being to limit appreciation of the people so labelled.

It is not, however, just dementia knowledge about which practitioners need to be critical. Being critical is not about criticising things or ideas. It is being willing and able to reflect on the advantages and disadvantages, to account for a number of different perspectives or arguments, and to make decisions from an informed position. Being a critical practitioner requires that you seek to learn, to not be satisfied with being subject to training, and it is an extension of the key activity that a relationship-centred approach to dementia care and support implies. The focus on learning suggests practitioners seek expertise from a variety of sources. At the core of their work, practitioners should be seeking to learn from three main sources.

The first is the person with dementia. If you recognise that the person with dementia is the expert in their own experiences of living life with dementia, then the reason for seeking to learn from this person is abundantly clear. Not seeking to do so will, in all likelihood, be because you have decided that this is not possible for you or because you do not believe that the person with dementia is capable of articulating their perspectives or views. A number of examples were given of persons with dementia speaking for themselves, *contributing to your knowledge* within these pages (see Chapter 2), as were organisations identified run by persons with dementia, for persons with dementia.

Questions about communication are not simply reducible to assessments of the level of impairment a person may have as a result of their dementia. You will not know what a person is capable of until you attempt genuinely to communicate with them. If, after trying a range of verbal and non-verbal approaches, communication proves impossible, then you must turn to other sources of knowledge and learning within the relationships you have in your role, in order to obtain what knowledge you can. The family member or supporter's perspective and knowledge become increasingly valuable in these circumstances. However, a person with dementia is a person, first and foremost, and has the right to have their views and perspectives listened to, heard and acted on. It is now established knowledge, and not news – persons with dementia can speak for themselves, until such point as they are unable to because of the impairments they experience. This point is not known in advance but discovered, over time, through interaction, during which communication must be presumed to continue and intelligence about the person recorded to enable information-sharing and possible future interpretation of behaviour and need.

The second of the three main sources of expertise is the family member or supporter. Along with seeking to learn from the person with dementia, the practitioner also needs to acknowledge the expertise of family members and supporters – and to learn from them, too. A better appreciation of their perspectives was encouraged with the use of the phrase 'walking in our footsteps'. Every family member or supporter will have a unique experience of dementia, and there are likely to be several people close to the person with dementia whose lives have been radically affected as a result. Who this includes is not immediately obvious and cannot be presumed. As a critical consumer of dementia knowledge, when listening to family members and supporters, the practitioner will not presume the popular rhetoric is true, that it is possible to 'live well with dementia'. It might not be.

What can be presumed, by reflecting on and learning from accounts provided by family members and supporters, are the kinds of feelings and expectations which these people might have when you meet them in your care and support settings. They continue to be in their own personal relationships with persons with dementia and these have been altered by dementia but remain as significant as any relationship *you* might have or have had with a loved one. Their desire to maintain and sustain these relationships while their loved one is cared for or supported by a practitioner must be respected and made as easy as possible. Practical obstacles to doing dementia care and support must not be allowed to blunt a sober appreciation of each family's enduring relationships.

Only by seeking to listen to family members and supporters is it possible to get a sense of who is affected and, in turn, what advice and information they might require to connect with appropriate local and national forms of support or services. Only by listening to these people will it also be possible to obtain rich and detailed biographical and preference information about the persons with dementia for whom you provide care or support. The quality of the relationship you develop with family members and supporters will determine how well you both do. Again, by seeking expertise from a variety of sources, engaging with and accessing your dementia care and support practice communities, you might learn and then share with family members and supporters the information and resources which they might require to meet their needs.

Approaching persons with dementia and family members and supporters as experts, seeking to learn from them, along with the additional responsibility and work of seeking expertise elsewhere, was summed up early in the book as taking the 'lead participant' role within relationship-centred dementia care. This 'status' is intended to put a name to the special responsibility that practitioners have within episodes of care and support, in those interactions overall, to lead this process. This lead responsibility already exists, of course, in terms of job or role, as a dementia care or support practitioner. 'Lead participant' is slightly different because 'participant' refers to the communication relationships that practitioners are a part of, and equal in, while undertaking their job or role.

By focusing on the communication relationships, rather than the specifics of role or job, it is hoped that the ideas associated with a critical, relationship-centred approach are applicable to all care and support practitioners. This is because they will all be characterised by the need to communicate with persons with dementia and their family members and supporters. What 'lead participant' status does, bringing with it all of the ideas contained within this book, is to drive not just what is done, but how it is done. *Doing* critical, relationship-centred dementia care and support is about taking the lead to ensure that communication occurs with those who have the expertise that practitioners need to do their job well but in ways (i.e. through learning and teaching) that mean everyone has their needs understood.

This is why I have described the role of dementia care and

support practitioners as pivotal, as involving leadership. And it is for this reason that the third source of expertise identified in this critical, relationship-centred approach is yours, the practitioner's. With so much appearing to hinge on the dementia care or support practitioner and the nature of their participation in communication relationships, it is only right to consider their experiences of dementia.

Rather than being considered to be without their own subjectivity or expertise, dementia care and support practitioners are viewed as human beings. It may seem a strange thing to claim but practitioners are often framed as simply 'care workers'. As 'care workers', they are expected to follow a range of guidelines and meet various expectations of what they should do and what they should know. This notion is utterly rejected. By exploring the experiences of dementia care and support practitioners, by giving practitioners respect for their thoughts, feelings, attitudes and knowledge, a number of important insights are gained about how and why dementia care and support is actually 'done' in practice. The 'care workers' narrative completely denies this complexity and, therefore, fails to capture and comprehend the reality of dementia care and support practice.

The private experience of dementia was identified as a range of influences which, typically, practitioners may not have cause to reveal. Yet, employing a variety of creative methods, it is possible to explore the formative events that shape individuals' choices to work with persons with dementia, touch on and discuss or communicate by other means their personal fears about dementia, and reflect on what it might mean to care for or support someone with dementia in ways practitioners might want for themselves. All of these insights are indicative, obtained from a very small number of practitioners. They are, however, really important if, as I do, you believe that interpersonal relationships are the beating heart of dementia care and support.

What it also does, this recognition of practitioners as human beings, is to provide a counter-argument to the way practitioners are often described dismissively as 'care workers'. Being a dementia care and support practitioner and *doing* dementia care and support is personal. When done well, it involves 'being with' persons with dementia and their family members and supporters – or, as Natasha Wilson put it, 'going there'. The insights practitioners provided about their private experiences of dementia demonstrate how seriously these individuals take their work – the passion to make a positive difference is a characteristic of many, if not all, accounts.

Yet these insights also lay bare the 'human resources' which underpin attempts to provide high-quality dementia care and support. In this recognition of the humanity of care and support practitioners, there needs also to be greater recognition of the support that should be made available to practitioners so that they are able to remain healthy and retain the high levels of motivation they have to do their work. The examples provided of practitioners being given access to 'art therapy'-type sessions should not, therefore, be viewed as outlandish or inappropriate. The stereotypes associated with those who care for and support persons with dementia as 'care workers' promote a view that anyone can do their work. This, I argue strongly, is absolutely not the case. It is possible that the greater visibility of and appreciation for the selfless work of NHS, care home and voluntary sector practitioners during the Covid-19 pandemic might lead to an overdue reassessment of pay for those working in dementia care and support. I have to be honest, I'm not confident it will. Yet, the proven worth of the proxy love and support given by so many practitioners to persons with dementia during these unprecedented times, in the absence of human contact with families and supporters, should be obvious for all to see. The thing is, dementia care and support practitioners undertake this kind of role in normal times, day in, day out. Maybe a way of showing your appreciation could be a letter to your MP suggesting improved pay and conditions for these 'care workers'?

Further recognition of the complexity and expertise of dementia care and support practitioners was provided with a focus on their practical experiences of dementia. This demonstrated that each practitioner possesses expertise about the way that dementia care and support is provided within their practice setting – including the barriers to improvement within their practice community, about which they are perfectly placed to offer intelligence. Examples of this practical knowledge, articulated by practitioners, were also shared. A focus on practical experience revealed that practitioners are members of wider groups of dementia practice communities, which possess further, collective expertise and resources. Practitioners were encouraged to think about how they engage with these communities and the kinds of actions they might take to improve dementia care and support by finding effective ways to communicate with their fellow practitioners.

Suggestions of an enhanced leadership role that practitioners might take by being proactive in these communities are qualified, as before, by pointing to the shared responsibility these practice communities have, as well as the organisations within which they are located. As has been noted, individual dementia care and support practitioners are not responsible for the overall quality of dementia care and support. Decisions about what action, if any, a practitioner takes must reflect what is feasible and practicable for that person. Drawing on and working with fellow practitioners in these communities of dementia care and support practice is the most effective way of seeking to bring about change or promote dialogue about an issue, problem or idea about dementia care or support practice. The mantra of 'do what you can do when you can do it' means doing so within these communities of practice.

To provide some inspiration for those looking to channel their commitment to dementia care and support into action, whatever the size of that action, the notion of the 'dementia passionista' was shared, along with ideas about the 'tribe' and 'going there'. Role models are important to anyone looking to develop and improve, and in dementia care and support there are very likely to be colleagues within communities of practice from whom practitioners could draw inspiration. The key is to become an active member of these communities. By doing so, it is more likely that practitioners will meet others with a similar drive and passion for the work that they do. And then, importantly, a practitioner will have an ally.

Other kinds of communities of practice were also identified: the 'dementia standards' communities. The point was made that practitioners have an obligation to know and understand the expectations for quality and standards of care within their settings. The argument was made for practitioners to take responsibility to discover what these standards for care and support are and, if necessary, share these with colleagues, who may not know them either. By making themselves fully aware of these standards, practitioners will become informed about the agreed benchmarks for service quality for their particular practice and also, if necessary, acquire a form of leverage for the suggestions they or their practice community might have for improvements.

A further point was made about membership of dementia standards communities. The suggestion was for dementia care and support practitioners to find ways to contribute their expertise to these communities. It was noted that dementia care and support practitioners could be under-represented in the groups which determine service and support standards. There is certainly a need for those with experiences of seeking to meet these standards in practice to be involved in determining standard setting. Ways of doing so were suggested to enable practitioners to have their voices and expertise heard and acted on. Not doing so, believing their knowledge is not valuable, amounts to accepting the current under-representation of frontline practitioners in care and support standard setting.

A similar argument was made for practitioners to pay attention to the dementia education standards communities, and view these as communities to which they are entitled full membership. It was argued that, again, dementia care and support practitioners – the primary intended audience of this book – do not appear to be adequately represented in decision-making groups which determine recommendations for practitioners' dementia knowledge. I have been invited to give my opinion and I'm not a dementia care or support practitioner. Have you? If not, this means that your expertise, your knowledge of what would really make a difference, is going unheard. Maybe it's time to cut out the middle-men and middle-women and have 'expertise' that originates primarily from talking to practitioners, to persons with dementia, and to family carers and supporters?

Some practitioners made it clear in their discussions about what I have called their practical experiences of dementia that both service standards and education are of tremendous value. How much more valuable would they be if they were better informed by practitioners' critical insight and expertise?

The critical, relationship-centred care and support approach is quite simple but, I hope, helpful in opening up thinking and discussion about the pivotal role of the dementia care and support practitioners and their sources of learning. With the suggestion that the person with dementia, the family member or supporter and the practitioner themselves have each a unique and valuable experience of dementia, the practitioner can orientate themselves towards learning. And, beyond the person with dementia the practitioner supports or cares for, there are various communities of persons with dementia from whom further learning can be undertaken. Similarly, beyond the family member or supporter, there are groups and communities representing family members and supporters from whom additional expertise can be accessed.

And, focusing on the individual practitioner, by following the direction of the relationships which you have with other practitioners, wider communities of dementia practice have been suggested, of which you are a member and within which you can engage. The *doing* of relationship-centred dementia care and support is suggested in the relationships you have, and by valuing those relationships and the expertise they connect. This includes your own expertise, your private and practical experiences of dementia. This is all premised, built on and sustained by the work you do, learning about others' experiences, making sense of this within the context of your own complex private and practical experiences of dementia, in the organisations for which you work. The passion you have for your work, with persons with dementia, their family members and supporters, is absolutely crucial. I hope that I have communicated adequately the high value in which it is regarded, not just by me, but by the persons with dementia and family members and supporters who have shaped the approach outlined in this book. This critical, relationship-centred approach to dementia care and support is intended to empower you in your work.

The passion and drive and commitment of dementia care and support practitioners must not be taken for granted but highly valued alongside a fairer, better rewarded and widely recognised expertise. At the centre of all discussions of excellence in dementia care and support are the people who do this work. The ideas presented in this book are intended to assist, alongside all the others that are available to you as a consumer of dementia knowledge. By using these ideas like lenses, you can see things and understand them in different ways. Having a repertoire of lenses at your disposal can only be of benefit to persons with dementia and their family members and supporters, as you strive towards excellence in your work and, in so doing, contribute to positive social change. Your commitment is to them, and not to ideas, models and theories.

It should be realised that whatever the aspirations for excellence in dementia, the 'standards' and 'recommendations', these are only as realistic and appropriate as the extent to which practitioners' expertise, and, yes, the call for more staffing and resources, are listened to. Organisations that deliver dementia care and support are each encouraged to consider creating their own 'University of Dementia'. This could be one positive step by which to begin to value, access, listen to and act on the dementia intelligence possessed by persons with dementia, family members and their supporters and dementia care and support practitioners. In turn, this would support and contribute to the underpinning relationship-centred basis of all dementia care and support, an approach which is, ultimately, personal to all involved.

I want to leave the last words to my inspirational friend, Colin Ward: 'The overriding thing I'd say is you've got to remember that everybody's different. Human beings are, generally speaking, all different. [Pause] Except for twins, maybe!' [Laughs]

References

Age UK (2020a) *Caring for Someone with Dementia*. Available at: www.ageuk.org.uk/information-advice/care/helping-a-loved-one/caring-dementia [Accessed 16/06/2020].

Age UK (2020b) *A New Milestone for Improving Dementia Care in Hospitals*. Available at: www.ageuk.org.uk/discover/2018/milestone-improving-dementia-care-in-hospitals [Accessed 06/08/2020].

All-Party Parliamentary Group on Dementia (2009) *Prepared to Care: Challenging the Dementia Skills Gap*. Available at: www.alzheimers.org.uk/sites/default/files/migrate/downloads/appg_report_prepared_to_care.pdf [Accessed 18/06/2020].

All-Party Parliamentary Group on Dementia (2013) *Dementia Does Not Discriminate: The Experiences of Black, Asian and Minority Ethnic Communities*. Available at: www.alzheimers.org.uk/sites/default/files/migrate/downloads/appg_2013_bame_report.pdf [Accessed 17/06/2020].

Alzheimer's Disease International (2020) *Early Symptoms*. Available at: www.alz.co.uk/info/early-symptoms [Accessed 10/05/2020].

Alzheimer's Research UK (2018) *Impact on Carers*. Available at: www.dementiastatistics.org/statistics/impact-on-carers [Accessed 16/06/2020].

Alzheimer's Research UK (2020) *Numbers of People in the UK*. Available at: www.dementiastatistics.org/statistics/numbers-of-people-in-the-uk [Accessed 17/05/2020].

Alzheimer's Society (2008) *Dementia: Out of the Shadows*. Available at: www.mentalhealth.org.uk/sites/default/files/out_of_the_shadows.pdf [Accessed 14/06/2020].

Alzheimer's Society (2016) *Fix Dementia Care: Hospitals*. Available at: www.alzheimers.org.uk/sites/default/files/migrate/downloads/fix_dementia_care_-_hospitals.pdf [Accessed 17/06/2020].

Alzheimer's Society (2018) *Positive Language: An Alzheimer's Society Guide to Talking About Dementia*. Available at: www.alzheimers.org.uk/sites/default/files/2018-09/Positive%20language%20guide_0.pdf [Accessed 14/06/2020].

Alzheimer's Society (2020a) *Types of Dementia*. Available at: www.alzheimers.org.uk/about-dementia/types-dementia [Accessed 10/05/2020].

Alzheimer's Society (2020b) *Young-Onset Dementia*. Available at: www.alzheimers.org.uk/about-dementia/types-dementia/younger-people-with-dementia [Accessed 17/05/2020].

Alzheimer's Society (2020c) *Dementia Talking Point*. Available at: https://forum.alzheimers.org.uk [Accessed 16/06/2020].

Alzheimer's Society (2020d) *This is Me: A Support Tool to Enable Person-Centred Care*. Available at: www.alzheimers.org.uk/get-support/publications-factsheets/this-is-me [Accessed 16/06/2020].

Bartlett, R. (2014) 'Citizenship in action: The lived experiences of citizens with dementia who campaign for social change.' *Disability & Society*, 29(8) 1291–1304.

Basting, A. (2018) 'Building creative communities of care: Arts, dementia, and hope in the United States.' *Dementia*, 17(6) 744–754.

Berrios, G.E. (1990) 'Alzheimer's disease: A conceptual history.' *International Journal of Geriatric Psychiatry*, 5, 355–365.

Brodaty, H. and Donkin, M. (2009) 'Family caregivers of people with dementia.' *Dialogues in Clinical Neuroscience*, 11(2) 217–228.

Cahill, S. (2018) *Dementia and Human Rights*. Bristol: Policy Press.

Care Quality Commission (2014) *Cracks in the Pathway: People's Experiences of Dementia Care as They Move Between Care Homes and Hospitals*. Available at: www.cqc.org.uk/sites/default/files/20141009_cracks_in_the_pathway_final_0.pdf [Accessed 17/06/2020].

Carers Trust (2020) *Resources*. Available at: https://carers.org/resources/all-resources?topic=%2CDementia+care&p=1 [Accessed 18/06/2020].

Carers UK (2020a) *Carers UK Forum*. Available at: www.carersuk.org/help-and-advice/get-support/carersuk-forum [Accessed 16/06/2020].

Carers UK (2020b) *Carer Passport Scheme*. Available at: www.carersuk.org/news-and-campaigns/campaigns/carer-passport-scheme [Accessed 16/06/2020].

Caring for the Carers (2020) *What are My Rights?* Available at: www.cftc.org.uk/resources-for-carers/what-are-my-rights [Accessed 16/06/2020].

Chambers Dictionary (2003) *Medicine* (ninth edition). London: John Murray Press.

Chambers Dictionary [online] (2020) *Syndrome.* Available at: https://chambers.co.uk/search/?query=syndrome&title=21st [Accessed 10/05/2020].

Chan, D., Livingston, G., Jones, L. and Sampson, E. (2013) 'Grief reactions in dementia carers: A systematic review.' *International Journal of Geriatric Psychiatry*, 28(1) 1–17.

Cohen, D. (1991) 'The subjective experience of Alzheimer's disease: The anatomy of an illness as perceived by patients and families.' *American Journal of Alzheimer's Care and Related Disorders and Research*, 6, 6–11.

Cohen, D. and Eisdorfer, C. (1986) *The Loss of Self: A Family Resource for the Care of Alzheimer's Disease and Related Disorders.* New York, NY: W.W. Norton.

Cooper, C., Marston, L., Barber, J., Livingston, D. *et al.* (2018) 'Do care homes deliver person-centred care? A cross-sectional survey of staff-reported abusive and positive behaviours towards residents from the MARQUE (Managing Agitation and Raising Quality of Life) English national care home survey.' *PLOS One*, 21 March 2018. Available at: https://doi.org/10.1371/journal.pone.0193399 [Accessed 21/06/2020].

Davis, R.L. (1989) *My Journey into Alzheimer's Disease.* Carol Stream, IL: Tyndale House Publishers.

Dementia Alliance International (2016) *The Human Rights of People Living with Dementia: From Rhetoric to Reality.* Available at: www.dementiaallianceinternational.org/wp-content/uploads/2016/04/The-Human-Rights-of-People-Living-with-Dementia-from-Rhetoric-to-Reality.pdf [Accessed 18/06/2020].

Dementia Alliance International (2017) *'Can You Hear Me Now?' by Carole Mullikan.* Available at: www.dementiaallianceinternational.org/tag/dasni [Accessed 14/06/2020].

Dementia Australia (2020) *Dementia Language Guidelines.* Available at: www.dementia.org.au/files/resources/dementia-language-guidelines.pdf [Accessed 14/06/2020].

Dementia Diaries (2020) Available at: https://dementiadiaries.org [Accessed 14/06/2020].

Dementia Engagement and Empowerment Project (2014) *Dementia Words Matter: Guidelines on Language about Dementia.* Available at: www.dementiavoices.org.uk/wp-content/uploads/2015/03/DEEP-Guide-Language.pdf [Accessed 14/06/2020].

Dementia Engagement and Empowerment Project (2020a) *About DEEP*. Available at: www.dementiavoices.org.uk [Accessed 14/06/2020].

Dementia Engagement and Empowerment Project (2020b) *Dementia Enquirers*. Available at: www.dementiavoices.org.uk/dementia-enquirers [Accessed 14/06/2020].

Dementia Engagement and Empowerment Project (2020c) *DEEP Guides for Organisations and Communities.* Available at: www.dementiavoices. org.uk/deep-guides/for-organisations-and-communities [Accessed 18/06/2020].

Dementia UK (2020a) *Types and Symptoms of Dementia.* Available at: www.dementiauk.org/understanding-dementia/types-and-symptoms [Accessed 10/05/2020].

Dementia UK (2020b) *Lewy Body Dementia.* Available at: www.dementiauk. org/understanding-dementia/types-and-symptoms/dementia-with-lewy-bodies [Accessed 10/05/2020].

Department of Health (2009) *Living Well with Dementia: A National Dementia Strategy.* Available at: www.gov.uk/government/uploads/ system/uploads/attachment_data/file/168220/dh_094051.pdf [Accessed 20/06/2020].

Department of Health (2015) *Prime Minister's Challenge on Dementia 2020.* Available at: https://assets.publishing.service.gov.uk/government/ uploads/system/uploads/attachment_data/file/414344/pm-dementia2020.pdf [Accessed 18/06/2020].

Dewing, J. (2006) 'Wandering into the future: Reconceptualizing wandering "a natural and good thing".' *International Journal of Older People Nursing,* 1(4) 239–249.

EDUCATE (2020) *Welcome to EDUCATE.* Available at: www. educatestockport.org.uk [Accessed 18/06/2020].

Friel McGowin, D. (1993) *Living in the Labyrinth: A Personal Journey Through the Maze of Alzheimer's.* New York, NY: Elder Books.

Gavan, J. (2011) 'Exploring the usefulness of a recovery-based approach to dementia care nursing.' *Contemporary Nurse,* 39(2) 140–146.

Gibson, F. (2004) *Past in the Present: Using Reminiscence in Health and Social Care.* Baltimore, MD: Health Professions Press.

Gilliard, J., Means, R., Beattie, A. and Daker-White, G. (2005) 'Dementia care in England and the social model of disability lessons and issues.' *Dementia,* 4(4) 571–586.

Golander, H. and Raz, A. (1996) 'The mask of dementia: Images of "demented residents" in a nursing home.' *Ageing and Society,* 16(5) 269–285.

Graham, J. and Bassett, R. (2006) 'Reciprocal relations: The recognition and co-construction of caring with Alzheimer's disease.' *Journal of Aging Studies*, 20(4) 335–349.

Greenwood, N., Mezey, G. and Smith, R. (2018) 'Social exclusion in adult informal carers: A systematic narrative review of the experiences of informal carers of people with dementia and mental illness.' *Maturitas*, 112, 39–45.

Greenwood, N. and Smith, R. (2019) 'Motivations for being informal carers of people living with dementia: A systematic review of qualitative literature.' *BMC Geriatrics*, 19, 169. Available at: https://doi.org/10.1186/s12877-019-1185-0 [Accessed 17/05/2020].

Guardian (2018) *Shops, Cafes and Round-the-Clock Care: Life in a 'Dementia Village'*. 12 March 2018. Available at: www.theguardian.com/society/shortcuts/2018/mar/12/life-dementia-village-development-kent-hogeweyk [Accessed 17/05/2020].

Guardian (2020a) *Tensions Rise over Race and Heritage as More Statues are Attacked*. 11 June 2020. Available at: www.theguardian.com/us-news/2020/jun/11/fears-of-violence-stop-london-racism-protest-as-statue-attacks-continue [Accessed 14/06/2020].

Guardian (2020b) *'We Did What We Set Out to Achieve': The Staff who Moved into Care Homes*. 28 April 2020. Available at: www.theguardian.com/society/2020/apr/28/we-did-what-we-set-out-to-achieve-the-staff-who-moved-into-care-homes [Accessed 16/06/2020].

Health, Social Services and Public Safety (2011) *Improving Dementia Services in Northern Ireland – A Regional Strategy*. Available at: www.health-ni.gov.uk/publications/improving-dementia-services-northern-ireland-regional-strategy [Accessed 17/06/2020].

Healthtalk.org (2018) *Carers of People with Dementia: Overview*. Available at: www.healthtalk.org/carers-people-dementia/overview [Accessed 16/06/2020].

Higher Education for Dementia Network (2013) *Curriculum for Dementia Education*. HEDN, Dementia UK. Available at: https://www.dementiauk.org/for-professionals/how-to-become-an-admiral-nurse/hedn [Accessed 16/09/2020].

Innovations in Dementia (2020) More information available at: www.innovationsindementia.org.uk [Accessed 19/06/2020].

Irish Times (2014) *Coming Out of the Shadows of Dementia*. 29 July 2014. Available at: www.irishtimes.com/life-and-style/the-health-centre/coming-out-of-the-shadows-of-dementia-1.1873415 [Accessed 14/06/2020].

Jeraj, S. and Butt, J. (2018) *Dementia and Black, Asian and Minority Ethnic Communities: Report of a Health and Wellbeing Alliance Project.* Available at: www.dementiaaction.org.uk/assets/0004/0379/Dementia_and_ BAME_Communities_report_Final_v2.pdf [Accessed 17/06/2020].

Johl, N., Patterson, T. and Pearson, L. (2016) 'What do we know about the attitudes, experiences and needs of Black and minority ethnic carers of people with dementia in the United Kingdom? A systematic review of empirical research findings.' *Dementia*, 15(4) 721–742.

John's Campaign (2020) Available at: https://johnscampaign.org.uk/# [Accessed 17/06/2020].

Killick, J. (1994) *Please Give Me Back My Personality! Writing and Dementia.* Stirling: Dementia Services Development Centre.

Kitwood, T. (1989) 'Brain, mind and dementia: With particular reference to Alzheimer's disease.' *Ageing & Society*, 9, 1–15.

Kitwood, T. (1990) 'The dialectics of dementia: With particular reference to Alzheimer's disease.' *Ageing & Society*, 10, 177–196.

Kitwood, T. (1993a) 'Person and process in dementia.' *International Journal of Geriatric Psychiatry*, 8, 541–545.

Kitwood, T. (1993b) 'Towards the Reconstruction of an Organic Mental Disorder.' In A. Radley (ed.) *Worlds of Illness*, pp.143–160. London: Routledge.

Kitwood, T. (1997a) *Dementia Reconsidered: The Person Comes First.* Buckinghamshire: Open University Press.

Kitwood, T. (1997b) 'The experience of dementia.' *Aging and Mental Health*, 1(1) 13–22.

Kitwood, T. and Bredin, K. (1992) 'Towards a theory of dementia care: Personhood and well-being.' *Ageing and Society*, 12, 269–287.

Leavey, G., Corry, D., Curren, E. and Waterhouse-Bradley, B. (2017) *Evaluation of a Healthcare Passport to Improve Quality of Care and Communication for People with Dementia* (EQuIP). Ulster University. Available at: https://research.hscni.net/sites/default/files/Evaluation%20 of%20a%20Healthcare%20Passport%20Brief%20report%207.6.18.pdf [Accessed 16/06/2020].

Lost Chord (2020) *Introduction.* Available at: https://lost-chord.co.uk [Accessed 17/06/2020].

Lyman, K.A. (1989) 'Bringing the social back in: A critique of the biomedicalization of dementia.' *Gerontologist*, 29(5) 597–605.

Maurer, K., Volk, S. and Gerbaldo, H. (1997) 'Auguste D and Alzheimer's disease.' *The Lancet*, 349, 1546–1549.

McKeown, J., Clarke, A., Ingleton, C., Ryan, T. and Repper, J. (2010) 'The use of life story work with people with dementia to enhance person-centred care.' *International Journal of Older People Nursing*, 5(2) 148–158.

Mead, G.H. (1934) *Mind, Self, and Society: From the Standpoint of a Social Behaviorist*. Chicago, IL: University of Chicago Press.

Merriam-Webster online (2020) *Biomedical*. Available at: www.merriam-webster.com/dictionary/biomedical [Accessed 17/05/2020].

Mitchell, W. (2018) *Somebody I Used to Know: A Memoir*. London: Bloomsbury Publishing.

Mobley, T. (2007) *Young Hope: The Broken Road*. Parker, CO: Outskirts Press.

Museums Association (2019) *Momentum Builds for Repatriation among UK Museums*. Available at: www.museumsassociation.org/museums-journal/news-analysis/12122019-momentum-for-repatriation-among-museums [Accessed 14/06/2020].

National Dementia Action Alliance (2019) *This Dementia Life. Episode 11: John L. Wood*. Available at: https://daanow.org/episode-11-john-l-wood [Accessed 15/06/2020].

National Dementia Action Alliance (2020) Available at: https://nationaldementiaaction.org.uk [Accessed 17/06/2020].

National Institute for Health and Care Excellence (2015) *Dementia, Disability and Frailty in Later Life – Mid-Life Approaches to Delay or Prevent Onset. NICE Guideline* [NG16]. Available at: www.nice.org.uk/guidance/ng16 [Accessed 18/06/2020].

National Institute for Health and Care Excellence (2018) *Dementia: Assessment, Management and Support for People Living with Dementia and their Carers. NICE Guideline* [NG97]. Available at: www.nice.org.uk/guidance/ng97 [Accessed 18/06/2020].

National Institute for Health and Care Excellence (2019) *Dementia Quality Standard [QS184]*. Available at: www.nice.org.uk/guidance/qs184 [Accessed 18/06/2020].

National Institute for Health and Care Excellence (2020a) *Improving Health and Social Care Through Evidence-Based Guidance*. Available at: www.nice.org.uk [Accessed 17/06/2020].

National Institute for Health and Care Excellence (2020b) *Guidance List: In Consultation*. Available at: www.nice.org.uk/guidance/inconsultation [Accessed 18/06/2020].

National Institute for Health and Care Excellence (2020c) *Get Involved*. Available at: www.nice.org.uk/get-involved [Accessed 18/06/2020].

National Institute for Health and Care Excellence (2020d) *Help Us Develop Quality Standards*. Available at: www.nice.org.uk/standards-and-indicators/get-involved [Accessed 18/06/2020].

National Institute for Health Research (2017) *Dementia Research – Colin & Irene's Story*. Available at: www.youtube.com/watch?v=4fETDi_-gDc [Accessed 15/06/2020].

National Institute for Health Research Involve (2020) *Briefing Notes for Researchers*. Available at: www.invo.org.uk/resource-centre/resource-for-researchers [Accessed 14/06/2020].

NHS (2019) *New Type of Dementia Identified*. Available at: www.nhs.uk/news/neurology/new-type-dementia-identified [Accessed 10/05/2020].

NHS England (2014) *Five Year Forward View*. Available at: www.england.nhs.uk/wp-content/uploads/2014/10/5yfv-web.pdf [Accessed 18/06/2020].

NHS England (2019) *NHS Hospitals Go Back to the Future for Dementia Care*. Available at: www.england.nhs.uk/2019/09/nhs-hospitals-go-back-to-the-future-for-dementia-care [Accessed 19/06/2020].

NHS England (2020) *Dementia*. Available at: www.england.nhs.uk/mental-health/dementia [Accessed 17/05/2020].

NHS Sheffield Clinical Commissioning Group (2019) *Sheffield Dementia Strategy Commitments: 2019–2024*. Available at: www.sheffieldccg.nhs.uk/Downloads/Our%20strategy/Mental%20Health%20etc/Sheffield%20Dementia%20Strategy%20Commitments.pdf [Accessed 18/06/2020].

Nolan, M., Ryan, T., Enderby, P. and Reid, D. (2002) 'Towards a more inclusive vision of dementia care practice and research.' *Dementia*, 1(2) 193–211.

O'Brien, C. (1996) 'Auguste D. and Alzheimer's disease.' *Science*, 273(5271) 28.

Oliver, M. (1990) *The Politics of Disablement*. London: Macmillan.

Page, S. and Fletcher, T. (2006) 'Auguste D. One hundred years on: "The person" not "the case".' *Dementia*, 5(4) 571–583.

Parliamentary and Health Service Ombudsman (2011) *Care and Compassion? Report of the Health Service Ombudsman on Ten Investigations into NHS Care of Older People*. London: The Stationery Office. Available at: www.ombudsman.org.uk/sites/default/files/2016-10/Care%20and%20Compassion.pdf [Accessed 17/05/2020].

Pham, T., Petersen, I., Walters, K., Raine, R. *et al.* (2018) 'Trends in dementia diagnosis rates in UK ethnic groups: Analysis of UK primary care data.' *Clinical Epidemiology*, 10, 949–960. Available at: www.ncbi.nlm.nih.gov/pmc/articles/PMC6087031 [Accessed 17/05/2020].

Playlist for Life (2019) *Connect with Friends and Family Through Music.* Available at: www.playlistforlife.org.uk [Accessed 17/06/2020].

Post, S.G. (2001) 'Comments on research in the social sciences pertaining to Alzheimer's disease: A more humble approach.' *Aging & Mental Health*, 5(S1) 17–19.

Pulsford, D., Hope, K. and Thompson, R. (2007) 'Higher education provision for professionals working with people with dementia: A scoping exercise.' *Nurse Education Today*, 27, 5–13.

Rare Dementia Support (2020) *Advice. Community. Learning.* Available at: www.raredementiasupport.org [Accessed 10/05/2020].

Reid, D. (1996) 'Methodology in Hearing the Voice of People with Dementia.' Unpublished MSc thesis, Department of Sociology & Social Policy, University of Stirling.

Reid, D. (1997) *'Who Knows the Person with Dementia?' Research in Progress.* 'Towards a social model of dementia'. Dementia Services Development Centre, Applied Social Science and Psychology Dementia Seminar Series, University of Stirling, 5 March.

Reid, D. (1998) *Who are People with Dementia? Acknowledging the Multiple Identities of Day Care Users Can Help Redefine Care Practice.* Presentation to the Society for the Study of Social Problems annual meeting, San Francisco, CA, August 1998.

Reid, D. (1999) *Conscience and Consent: Involving People with Dementia in Social Research.* Presentation to the Society for the Study of Social Problems annual meeting, Chicago, IL, August 1999.

Reid, D. (2009a) *The National Dementia Strategy Objective 13: Time for a Dialogue Between Education and Training.* British Society of Gerontology Annual Conference, UWE, 1–3 September.

Reid, D. (2009b) *Teaching Dementia Care Skills: Moving Beyond a Competency-Based Approach.* Global Connections International Nursing Symposium, King Faisal Specialist Hospital, Riyadh, Saudi Arabia, 27–28 October.

Reid, D. (2014) 'An annual offer of creative "here and now" moments.' *The Journal of Dementia Care*, 22(3) 24–27.

Reid, D. (2019) *Sheffield Dementia Information Pack.* Available at: https://sydcae.co.uk/SDIP-November-2019.pdf [Accessed 21/06/2020].

Reid, D., Ryan, T. and Enderby, P. (2001) 'What does it mean to listen to people with dementia?' *Disability and Society*, 16(3) 377–392.

Reid, D., Warnes, T. and Low, L. (2014) '"Living well...I like the sound of that".' *The Journal of Dementia Care*, 22(1) 29–31.

Reid, D. and Witherspoon, R. (2008) *Dementia Essentials: The Development of a Foundation Course in Dementia Education*. Paper presentation at Dementia Congress, Bournemouth, November 2008.

Research England (2020) *REF Impact*. Available at: https://re.ukri.org/research/ref-impact [Accessed 15/06/2020].

Research Excellence Framework (2014) *REF2014 Impact Case Studies*. Available at: https://impact.ref.ac.uk/casestudies/FAQ.aspx [Accessed 15/06/2020].

Rose, L. (1996) *Show Me the Way to Go Home*. New York, NY: Elder Books.

Royal Surgical Aid Society (2016) *The Experiences, Needs and Outcomes for Carers of People with Dementia: Literature Review*. Available at: https://dementiacarers.org.uk/wp-content/uploads/2018/11/RSAS-ADS-Experiences-needs-outcomes-for-carers-of-people-with-dementia-Lit-review-2016.pdf [Accessed 16/06/2020].

Ryan, T., Nolan, M., Enderby, P. and Reid, D. (2004) '"Part of the family": Sources of job satisfaction among a group of community-based dementia care workers.' *Health & Social Care in the Community*, 12 (2) 111–118.

Ryan, T., Nolan, M., Reid, D. and Enderby, P. (2008) 'Using the Senses Framework to achieve relationship-centred dementia care services: A case example.' *Dementia*, 7, 71–93.

Sabat, S. (2001) *The Experience of Alzheimer's Disease: Life Through a Tangled Veil*. Oxford: Blackwell Publishers.

Sabat, S.R. and Harrè, R. (1992) 'The construction and deconstruction of self in Alzheimer's disease.' *Ageing & Society*, 12, 443–461.

Schweitzer, P. and Bruce, E. (2008) *Remembering Yesterday, Caring Today. Reminiscence in Dementia Care: A Guide to Good Practice*. London: Jessica Kingsley Publishers.

Scottish Government (2017) *Scotland's National Dementia Strategy 2017–2020*. Available at: www.gov.scot/binaries/content/documents/govscot/publications/strategy-plan/2017/06/scotlands-national-dementia-strategy-2017-2020/documents/00521773-pdf/00521773-pdf/govscot%3Adocument/00521773.pdf [Accessed 17/06/2020].

Seattle Times (2018) *Let's Talk about Dementia to Bring It Out of the Shadows*. Available at: www.seattletimes.com/opinion/lets-talk-about-dementia-to-bring-it-out-of-the-shadows [Accessed 14/06/2020].

Sheffield Dementia Involvement Group (2020) *Sheffield Dementia Involvement Group (SHINDIG)*. Available at: www.shsc.nhs.uk/get-involved/service-user-groups/sheffield-dementia-involvement-group-shindig [Accessed 18/06/2020].

Sheffield Health and Social Care NHS Foundation Trust and the Alzheimer's Society Sheffield (2013) *The Voice of Dementia*. Available at: https://vimeo.com/57843638 [Accessed 14/06/2020].

Sikes, P. (2020) Personal communication (22/06/2020).

Sikes, P. and Hall, M. (2018) "'It was then that I thought "whaat? This is not my Dad": The implications of the "still the same person" narrative for children and young people who have a parent with dementia.' *Dementia*, 17(2) 180–198.

Skills for Care & Skills for Health (2011) *Common Core Principles for Supporting People with Dementia – A Guide to Training the Social Care and Health Workforce*. Available at: www.skillsforcare.org.uk/Document-library/Skills/Dementia/CCP-Dementia-(webv2)%5B1%5D.pdf [Accessed 20/06/2020].

Skills for Health, Skills for Care and Health Education England (2015) *Dementia Core Skills Education and Training Framework*. Available at: www.skillsforhealth.org.uk/images/projects/dementia/Dementia%20Core%20Skills%20Education%20and%20Training%20Framework.pdf [Accessed 19/06/2020].

Skills for Health, Skills for Care and Health Education England (2018) *Dementia Training Standards Framework*. Available at: www.hee.nhs.uk/our-work/dementia-awareness/core-skills [Accessed 17/06/2020].

Social Care Institute for Excellence (2015a) *Dementia-Like Symptoms: What Else Could It Be?* Available at: www.scie.org.uk/dementia/symptoms/diagnosis/what-else.asp [Accessed 10/05/2020].

Social Care Institute for Excellence (2015b) *Becoming the Carer of a Person with Dementia*. Available at: www.scie.org.uk/dementia/carers-of-people-with-dementia/working-in-partnership/becoming-a-carer.asp [Accessed 16/06/2020].

Social Care Institute for Excellence (2019) *Dementia Awareness E-Learning Course*. Available at: www.scie.org.uk/e-learning/dementia [Accessed 16/06/2020].

Social Care Institute for Excellence (2020) *Dementia: At a Glance*. Available at: www.scie.org.uk/dementia/about [Accessed 17/05/2020].

Southern Health NHS Foundation Trust (2019) *Dementia Services*. Available at: www.southernhealth.nhs.uk/services/mental-health/specialist-mental-health-services/dementia-service [Accessed 06/08/2020].

South Yorkshire Dementia Creative Arts Exhibition (SYDCAE) (2020) *South Yorkshire Dementia Creative Arts Exhibition*. Available at: www.sydcae.co.uk [Accessed 17/06/2020].

Stelzmann, R.A., Schnitzlein, H.N. and Murtagh, F.R. (1995) 'An English translation of Alzheimer's 1907 paper, "Über eine eigenartige Erkrankung der Hirnrinde"'. *Clinical Anatomy*, 8, 429–431.

Stokes, G. (2017) *Challenging Behaviour in Dementia: A Person-Centred Approach*. Oxford: Routledge.

Surr, C., Baillie, L., Waugh, A. and Brown, M. (2016) *Position Paper: The Importance of Including Dementia in Pre- and Post-Registration Curricula for Health and Social Care Professionals. Draft 1 – Not for Circulation*. Received as member of the Higher Education for Dementia Network (HEDN).

Surr, C. and Gates, C. (2016) *What Works in Dementia Training and Education?* PowerPoint presentation. Available at: www.careinfo.org/wp-content/uploads/2016/11/The-What-Works-study-Claire-Surr-and-Cara-Gates-Leeds-Beckett-University.pdf [Accessed 15/03/2017].

Surr, C., Gates, C., Irving, D., Oyebode, J. *et al.* (2016) *What Works in Dementia Training and Education? A Critical Interpretive Synthesis of the Evidence*. Poster available at: www.heacademy.ac.uk/system/files/downloads/surr_what_works_in_dementia_training.pdf [Accessed 19/06/2020].

Swaffer, K. (2016) *What the Hell Happened to my Brain? Living Beyond Dementia*. London: Jessica Kingsley Publishers.

The Francis Report (2013) *Report of the Mid Staffordshire NHS Foundation Trust Public Inquiry: Executive Summary*. Available at: https://assets.publishing.service.gov.uk/government/uploads/system/uploads/attachment_data/file/279124/0947.pdf [Accessed 17/05/2020].

The National Archives (2020) *How to Look for Records of Asylums, Psychiatric Hospitals and Mental Health*. Available at: www.nationalarchives.gov.uk/help-with-your-research/research-guides/mental-health [Accessed 14/06/2020].

Tresolini, C.P. and the Pew-Fetzer Task Force (1994) *Health Professions Education and Relationship-Centered Care*. San Francisco, CA: Pew Health Professions Commission.

Tsaroucha, A., Benbow, S.M., Kingston, P. and Le Mesurier, N. (2011) 'Dementia skills for all: A core competency framework for the workforce in the United Kingdom'. *Dementia*, 12(1) 29–44.

Usher, K.J. and Arthur, D. (1998) 'Process consent: A model for enhancing informed consent in mental health nursing'. *Journal of Advanced Nursing*, 27, 692–697.

Vittoria, A.K. (1998) 'Preserving selves: Identity work and dementia'. *Research on Aging*, 20(1) 91–136.

Welsh Government (2018) *Dementia Action Plan for Wales 2018–2022.* Available at: https://gov.wales/sites/default/files/publications/2019-04/dementia-action-plan-for-wales.pdf [Accessed 17/06/2020].

Wood, J. (2020) *Sculpture.* Available at: www.johnlouiswood.com/home.html [Accessed 15/05/2020].

Wood, J., Reid, D. and Marks, K. (2016) 'University of Dementia.' In *Facing Outwards: Engaged Learning at the University of Sheffield* (pp.36–38). Available at: www.sheffield.ac.uk/polopoly_fs/1.661883!/file/FacingOutwards.pdf [Accessed 19/06/2020].

Woods, R.T. (1989) *Alzheimer's Disease: Coping with a Living Death.* London: Souvenir Press.

YoungDementia UK (2019) *Support and Friendship Online.* Available at: www.youngdementiauk.org/support-friendship-online [Accessed 16/06/2020].

YoungDementia UK (2020) *Living with a Learning Disability and Young Onset Dementia.* Available at: www.youngdementiauk.org/blogs/living-learning-disability-and-young-onset-dementia [Accessed 19/06/2020].

Author Biography

David Reid is the director of DARE Dementia, a community interest company, aimed at supporting persons with dementia and their supporters to enjoy an enhanced quality of life. David has previously worked as a development worker for a large UK-based dementia charity and spent nearly 20 years working in higher education as a researcher, lecturer and university teacher. He has contributed to academic publications on relationship-centred dementia care and written and led dementia education courses up to master's degree level. David also founded and continues to lead the annual South Yorkshire Dementia Creative Arts Exhibition.

Subject Index

academic research
  focus of 50-1
  generalisations in 49
acceptance 22, 26
advice
  for family members 86-7, 156
  from persons with dementia 56-8
age and dementia (assumptions about) 24-5
anticipatory grief 76
appropriation 41-2
art therapy sessions 123-36
arts *see* creative arts
autobiographical works 41, 43-4

barriers identified by practitioners 102-4
biomedical approach
  definition of 20-1
  dehumanizing gaze of 39
  dominance of 22
  questioning the claims of 20-1, 24, 46
boundaries 153

care practitioner *see* dementia care practitioner
Carer Passport Scheme 80, 81
carers' rights 79

see also family members and supporters
clinical setting 101-2
communication
  with person with dementia 187
  poems (John Killick) 44
  quality of (lead participant) 91-2
communities (practice) 155-62
core competencies 173-4
Covid-19 pandemic 191-2
creative arts
  art therapy sessions 123-36
  drawing exercise 120-3
  exhibitions 36, 58-9
  music 139-42
credit (to persons with dementia) 43, 48-9
critical approach to knowledge 15, 29-30
critical thought 92
cultural influences 119

day-care services (learning in) 52-5
'defeating dementia' (concept of) 22
dementia
  as syndrome 23
  as a term of convenience 23-5
  see also person with dementia
Dementia Action Plan (Wales) 160

Author Index